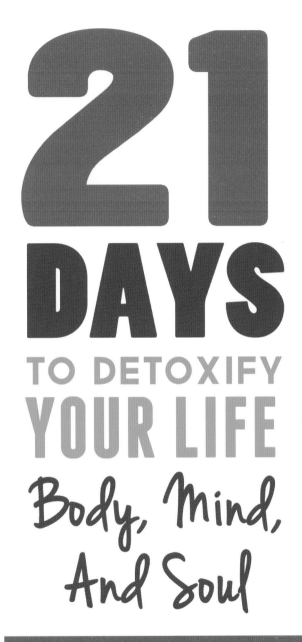

21 DAYS
TO DETOXIFY
YOUR LIFE

Body, Mind, And Soul

ADELE CAVALIERE

Logan Hocking County
District Library
230 East Main Street
Logan, Ohio 43138

D1404631

Front Table Books   An Imprint of Cedar Fort, Inc.   Springville, Utah

© 2014 Adele Cavaliere
All rights reserved.

No part of this book may be reproduced in any form whatsoever, whether by graphic, visual, electronic, film, microfilm, tape recording, or any other means, without prior written permission of the publisher, except in the case of brief passages embodied in critical reviews and articles.

ISBN: 978-1-4621-1525-9

Published by Front Table Books, an imprint of Cedar Fort, Inc.
2373 W. 700 S., Springville, UT, 84663
Distributed by Cedar Fort, Inc., www.cedarfort.com

LIBRARY OF CONGRESS CATALOGING-IN-PUBLICATION DATA
  Cavaliere, Adele, 1980-
  21 days to detoxify your life / Adele Cavaliere.
    pages cm
  ISBN 978-1-4621-1525-9
  1. Detoxification (Health) 2. Nutrition. 3. Exercise. 4. Reducing diets. I. Title. II.
  Title: Twenty one days to detoxify your life.
  RA784.5.C38 2014
  613--dc23
                   2014026877

Cover and page design by Bekah Claussen
Cover design © 2014 by Lyle Mortimer
Edited by Hannah Ballard and Rachel Munk

Printed in China

1 2 3 4 5 6 7 8 9 10

ARE YOU READY:

to watch your energy levels soar,
cleanse your body of harmful toxins,
give your skin a healthy glow,
gain unparalleled mental clarity,
and even lose those unwanted pounds
along the way?

**THEN COME WITH ME
ON THIS AMAZING JOURNEY
OF DETOXIFICATION
FROM THE INSIDE-OUT!**

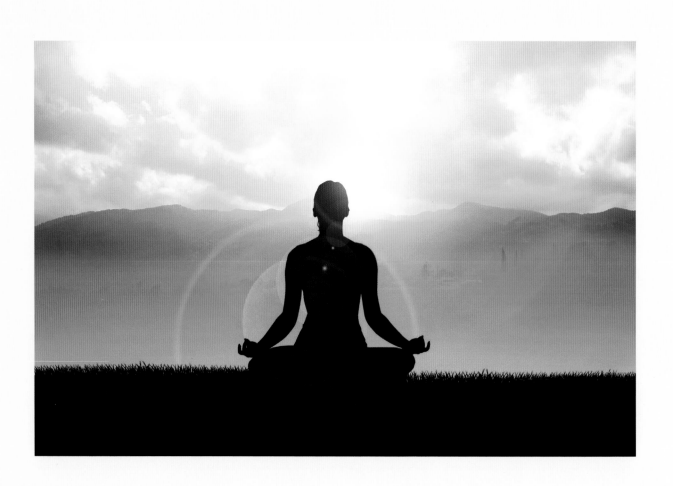

CONTENTS

I AM ADELE CAVALIERE, FOUNDER OF METABODY INC., CELEBRITY NUTRITIONIST, ELITE FITNESS TRAINER, CERTIFIED LIFE AND WELLNESS COACH, AND YOUR PARTNER IN CHANGE.

When I sat down to create this program, I had one thought in mind: to share all the incredible things I've learned over the years about the power of cleansing, and to help others who, like me, want to find their path to perfect health and a life filled with vitality, joy, and positivity. Over the next 21 days, I am going to help you reclaim your health and transform your life in ways you may not have even thought possible.

Many of us have a complicated relationship with food, made even more complicated by its necessity. And it is necessary that you start to understand your relationship with food before starting this program. Take a moment now to ask yourself a few questions: What types of food are you drawn to? Do you eat out of boredom or another emotional state? Are you using food to fill up other areas that feel empty? Taking the time to understand the connections between you and your food is an important step in recognizing negative patterns and taking the appropriate action to change them, while building a better relationship with your mind and your body—something you will achieve over the course of the next 21 days.

In fact, the very act of cleansing opens up the lines of communication between you and your body, allowing for a deeper understanding of what it needs and how to listen to what it's telling you. For example, cravings can be your body's way of letting you know it needs something. But since many North Americans consistently feed their bodies high-sugar, over-processed foods, their bodies have been programmed to crave only those foods. The purpose of a detox is to reset your palate so that you no longer experience these types of "bad" cravings and instead

return your body to a mainly "non-craving" state. Furthermore, the ability to tune into the physical signs your body gives you when something is amiss will allow you to diagnose the problem (whether it is a congested liver or clogged kidneys) and take action to remedy it on your own.

Feeling a little overwhelmed? Don't worry. Over the course of the program, we will explore these topics together, and by the end you will be the expert on your own body!

And on that note—let's get back to the program! Over the next 21 days, I am going to show you how making small changes can have a big impact on your overall health. Each day I will ask you to incorporate a simple change to your eating habits, add some light activity to your daily routine, or expand your mind and help you reach a sense of inner peace through a life coaching or meditation exercise. Though the changes will be small, they are realistic and sustainable, and can have a big effect on your overall health while preparing you for bigger changes down the road.

This journey will be thoroughly educational. You will not only learn about your body, how it works, and how to keep it running at its best, but you will also learn how to embrace a whole new way of living while taking responsibility for yourself. You'll learn to live the vital and empowered kind of life you know you deserve, not just today, but for the rest of your life!

Starting any new diet plan can seem daunting since it involves change, and change can be a scary thing! But when we embrace it with our whole hearts, anything becomes possible. We all have the power to change inside of us. We just need to find the inspiration to ignite it. I always tell my clients: "The first love is self-love." Loving yourself means wanting the best for yourself. And the best part is that when you give love to yourself, you're better able to give love to others. It's like a love ripple effect! So you see, when making positive changes to your own life, you in effect make positive changes in the lives of the ones you love. Pretty amazing, huh?

It's true that we live in a busy world with schedules, deadlines, and seemingly endless obligations. But if you start small, you can make important changes that can have a big impact while giving you the momentum to make even bigger changes until you reach your goals. Each day, commit to making a small change, like cutting sugar from your diet (it really is white poison), walking to the grocery store instead of driving, or taking 15 minutes to sit quietly by yourself and breathe deeply. It won't be long before you'll notice how much better you feel, how much more glowing your skin looks, or how much more calm and at peace you feel. Make this commitment to yourself today and tomorrow is already a little brighter. This is my promise to you.

So, without further ado . . . let's get detoxifying!

Your partner in change,

Adele Cavaliere

Adele Fridman is a celebrity nutritionist, elite trainer, certified life coach, sports nutrition teacher for the Canadian School of Natural Nutrition, and the founder of MetaBody Inc., Nutri-Wellness Inc., and Nutri-school. But this dynamic woman, mom, entrepreneur, and fitness guru is also so much more.

Like many, Adele's story of transformation began when after years of struggling with personal challenges she found herself overweight, depressed, lethargic, and unable to recognize the woman she had become. Determined to unleash the extraordinary woman she knew still existed inside her, Adele made the decision to change her life and embrace the future she knew she deserved. And she wasn't going to do it alone.

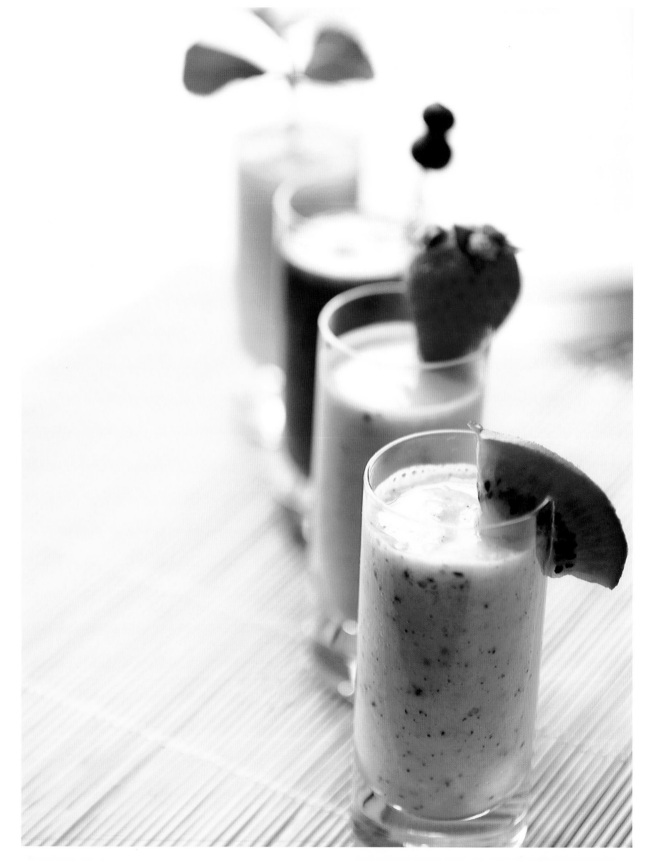

GETTING PREPPED AND PACKED FOR THE JOURNEY

Before we set off on this amazing adventure of personal transformation, we need to get make sure we're ready. In my experience, detox programs are fun and easy, as long as you start with the right attitude and the right prep! Before we get into the program, I want to take you through the best ways to prepare your body, your mind, and your kitchen for this journey. After all, you wouldn't climb a mountain without a map and the right equipment, would you? Heck, no!

So let's start with a few helpful pre-program actions you can take to help ease yourself into "detox" mode while giving you the proper start needed to ensure a strong finish!

PURGE THAT PANTRY!

Unless you possess superhuman self-control, it can be difficult to resist the call of junk food coming from your cupboard. To help avoid temptation, I recommend that all clients begin a detox by cleansing their pantry and fridge of all the processed, sugary, and fat-laden foods that could hinder their success. After all, you can't eat what's not there! Don't worry, we will be filling it right back up with delicious and nutritious foods that not only taste great, but that are also going to help give your body and mind the overhaul they need.

DE-CLUTTER THE FENG SHUI WAY

We North Americans seem to have an obsession with stuff, often filling our homes and office spaces with things we simply don't need. But research has shown that a cluttered space leads to increased stress, mental chaos, and feelings of anxiety and loss of control. This is why, before starting this program, I recommend that you take the time to cleanse your environment and set the stage for a fresh, positive, and more relaxed way of living. And because de-cluttering a room offers immediate and clear results, you start to feel the positive effects straight away, motivating you to continue on to bigger goals. Here are a few quick tips to help you get started:

Start small, even if it's only with a single drawer or cupboard.

Make de-cluttering a quick 15-minute weekly routine.

Get in the habit of putting things away immediately rather than doing it later.

Store away seldom used items and dispose or donate unused ones.

Use plenty of containers when storing items and label containers when necessary.

Enlist the help of friends. They aren't as attached to your things as you are.

Teach your family to be responsible for their mess.

Address the emotional reasons why you collect clutter.

Don't forget about important spaces outside the home, such as your office and your car.

Looking to get that positive energy flowing even more? How about a little feng shui! Feng shui is a Chinese system of geomancy that uses the laws of both Heaven and Earth to help one improve life by receiving positive qi (or life force). The principles can be pretty complex, but I think many of us would love for our homes to feel more restful and at peace. Luckily, it's a cinch to start working simple feng shui practices into your life. Here are a few simple room-by-room ways to feng shui your home and start benefiting from those positive vibes!

YOUR BEDROOM

Position your bed within view of the door and windows, close off the closet and bathroom, and avoid hanging anything heavy over the bed.

YOUR DESK

Make sure you are facing the door so you can accept positive energy. Keep your desk neat and tidy, and try incorporating purple—an energizing color—around your space. While this may seem surprising, the color black is great for careers and money, and also promotes creativity. Don't forget flowers or houseplants. Also include a few personal mementos to connect you to those you love—it will promote an energized and more focused mind set while working.

YOUR CLOSET

An organized closet works wonders in not only allowing you to fully utilize storage space in a small home or condo, but it also has a great effect on helping you feel more settled in your bedroom. Closets

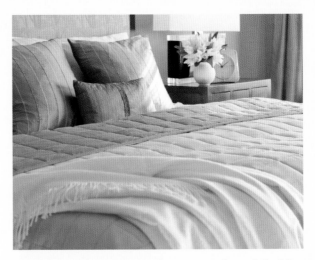

should be neat, tidy, well organized, and hidden behind doors. Try leaving empty space to promote the flow of energy.

YOUR LIVING ROOM

Your living room should be warm, inviting, and a reflection of your personal style. Include artwork, photos, and family heirlooms to welcome others into your space. Opt for as much natural lighting as possible and avoid overhead lighting, which can make the energy feel too harsh. Also, choosing a lighter color for the walls can help the space seem brighter and more open.

YOUR KITCHEN

Not only is it much easier to cook in a kitchen that is neat and orderly, but it also helps the positive energy flow freely and straight into your food as you cook! Introduce energizing colors, greenery, or plants to add life to the room. You should feel like the captain of your kitchen, so try to arrange it so you face the entryway while you cook. If this isn't possible, hanging a mirror or other reflective item over the stove can help redirect energy.

START YOUR FOOD DIARY

In the introduction of this program, I touched on the importance of understanding your relationship with food. One of the most effective ways to do this is by keeping a food journal, in which you keep track of not only what you eat, but also what you'd *like* to eat (your cravings) and whether or not you give in to those cravings. Also, track when you eat and if there was any emotional reason behind the eating. Often we forget about the odd treat here or there, are simply oblivious to how we eat on a daily basis, or fail to make the connection behind our motivation to eat (for example, boredom). Writing it down puts it all out there for you in black and white. And once you understand your relationship with food, you can begin to repair and change it.

Before starting the program, keep a 3-day food journal and write down what you eat, when you eat, and how you felt that day.

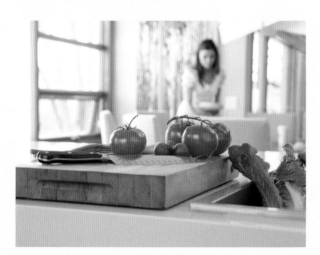

Here is an example of how an entry might look:

MONDAY

Time: *8 AM*

Location: *At the kitchen table, at my desk, and so on.*

What were you doing?
Reading the paper/checking my email/and so on.

Meal included: *2 scrambled eggs, 1 slice brown toast with jam, and so on.*

How were you feeling physically?
Slight headache/sore back/and so on.

How were you feeling mentally?
Feeling slightly down/anxious about a meeting/and so on.

When you look back over your day, you may find that some of your mental and physical feelings were a result of what you were eating. You may also discover that you are not eating at the right times for your body, or at the right frequency. If you find you are hungry and have low energy in the afternoon between lunch and dinner, you may want to break up those larger meals into three smaller meals, one being consumed in the mid-afternoon. Study your findings and learn to listen to your body. As you gain more knowledge about your eating habits and what your body needs, choosing the right foods will become second nature.

TAKE BODY MEASUREMENTS

I know this might be a discouraging task, but it is necessary in understanding where you are now physically and the change you will see moving forward. And with the right commitment, you *will* see change. Remember that you are at the beginning of your journey. Be proud that you're making this commitment today!

Here is a quick guide on how to take proper measurements:

Waist: Without holding the tape too tight, measure the narrowest part of your trunk, approximately 1 inch above your belly button.

Hips: Measure around the fullest part of your buttocks with your heels together.

Thighs: Measure the upper thighs, just below where the buttocks merge with the back thigh.

Chest: Measure around the fullest part of the chest.

Once you have taken your body measurements, you will need to weigh yourself and calculate your body fat percentage. The best time to do this is first thing in the morning after you have gone to the bathroom. Many consumer scales today have Bio-electric Impedence Analysis or BIA capabilities, that measure body fat by determining the electrical impedance, or opposition to the flow of an electric current, through the body. I recommend making a small investment and purchasing one. It will not only come in handy over the next 21 days, but in all the days after.

Lastly, you will also need to take a before photo at this time to be used to track your progress. This might also be a daunting task, but try not to feel embarrassed or ashamed of how you look now. Get empowered by the action you are taking today, and work that camera!

IT ALL STARTS IN THE GUT

No matter what diet or nutritional lifestyle you subscribe to, one thing remains true for everyone: as humans, we truly are what we eat. If we feed our bodies wholesome, nutrient-rich foods, they flourish, giving us the energy and good health needed to live a long, vital, and active life. But if we feed our bodies what I call "non-foods," foods that contain no nutritional value and only empty calories, we not only rob ourselves of the powerful life we could be living, but we also put ourselves at risk of suffering serious health problems. And it all starts with your digestive system.

Here's a quick health studies lesson. Digestion is the means by which our bodies extract nutrients from our food to use as energy in order to function. It begins the minute we start chewing our food. Food is partly broken down by the process of chewing and partly by the chemical action of salivary enzymes. Once we've enjoyed the bite of whatever we're munching on, we swallow, pushing the food down to our stomach where is it churned and bathed in a strong acid called gastric acid. Once the stomach is finished doing its thing, food moves to the small intestine where bile (produced in the liver and stored in the gall bladder), pancreatic enzymes, and other digestive enzymes produced by the inner wall of the small intestine help in the breakdown of food. From there, it travels to the large intestine where some of the water and electrolytes (chemicals like sodium) are removed from the food. Many microbes (bacteria like Bacteroides, Lactobacillus acidophilus, Escherichia coli, and Klebsiella) in the large intestine help in the digestion process. Food then travels through the colon and out of your body. And all the while, the body is absorbing the crucial nutrients it needs to fight disease; manage your body's heart, nerve, and muscle functions; regulate the production and use of hormones in your endocrine system; keep your body fluids balanced; and support your metabolism.

Poor digestion leaves the body with a lack of nutritional factors to support proper immune functioning, as well as the functioning of the body as a whole. This is because a poorly functioning digestive system has lost some of its ability to break down our food and extract and absorb the nutrients the body needs to run. To compensate, an inadequate digestive system will steal enzymes from the immune system to operate, therefore weakening immune function and making the body more vulnerable to disease.

The recipe for proper digestion is a diet of whole, unprocessed foods that are not only filled with the vitamins and nutrients our bodies need, but also work to eliminate the harmful toxins that are negatively affecting our digestion.

DETOX AND CLEANSE DIETS
WHAT THE HECK DO THEY REALLY DO?

Unlike our ancestors, we are constantly bombarded with toxins. Found everywhere from the air we breathe to the food we eat to the products we put on our skin, our bodies are forced to work overtime to cope with these toxic foreign invaders while our health, both physical and mental, suffers greatly. The purpose of a detox or cleanse is to remove these toxins from our bodies and bring it back into a balanced state.

Now here comes the warning that I am about to get a little "high school science class" on you, but understanding your body and how it functions is key to achieving optimal health.

You've most likely heard the term "pH levels" in relation to how certain soaps can be drying to your skin, but the importance of pH levels goes far beyond the choice between Dove and Irish Spring. When we talk about the natural PH levels in our bodies, we are really discussing how acid or alkaline our cells are. We run best when our cells are slightly alkaline, therefore we want to avoid foods that are acid-forming, which make us susceptible to diseases, like cancer, by damaging our cells.

Unfortunately, the typical North American's diet is riddled with acid-forming foods, such as over-processed meats, dairy, sugar, coffee, alcohol, and pretty much anything that comes in a can or box. A detox seeks to bring the body back to its slightly alkaline state by eliminating these acidic foods and replacing them with naturally cleansing, whole, alkaline-forming foods.

ACID- AND ALKALI-FORMING FOODS

As mentioned earlier, one big problem afflicting North Americans is their highly acid-forming diets. Chocolate, alcohol, cakes, crackers, sugar, red meat—these common acid forming foods wreak havoc in our bodies. You see, when we eat, a sort of ash is created as a by-product of digestion. When this ash is alkaline or neutral, it can be easily swept up without leaving behind any harsh residue. But if the ash is highly acidic (the body can handle a small dose of acids), then this residue builds and your body cannot cope, causing it to become unbalanced and toxic.

Common symptoms of acidosis include weight gain, fatigue, headaches, skin rashes and disorders, osteoporosis, and too many other issues to mention here.

But don't worry, this situation can be reversed, and quite easily! All you have to do is rebalance your body by introducing a diet of alkali-forming foods and you'll be basking in the glow of your skin, the bounce in your step, and the general air of well-being surrounding you.

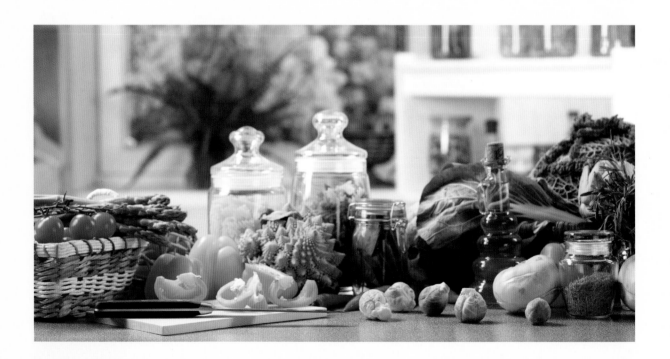

Here are some common acid-forming and alkali-forming foods:

ALKALI FORMING

» Alfalfa	» Peppers	» Almonds
» Broccoli	» Spinach	» Millet
» Carrots	» Sweet Potatoes	» Whey Protein Powder
» Cauliflower	» Tomatoes	» Cinnamon
» Celery	» Apples	» Curry
» Chard Greens	» Avocados	» Ginger
» Garlic	» Berries	» Herbs (all)

ACID FORMING

» Corn	» Rice (all)	» Beef
» Lentils	» Rice Cakes	» Pork
» Olives	» Rye	» Tuna
» Winter Squash	» Black Beans	» Turkey
» Blueberries	» Chickpeas	» Olive Oil
» Bread	» Cheese	
» Quinoa	» Peanuts	

Because our bodies are an alkaline entity, in order to maintain health, the majority of our diet must consist of alkaline foods. We can remain in good health by consuming a diet that is 70–80% alkaline and 20–30% acid.

It is important to note that a food's acid- or alkaline-forming tendency in the body has nothing to do with the actual pH of the food itself. For example, lemons are very acidic; however, the end products they produce after digestion and assimilation are very alkaline, so lemons are alkali-forming in the body. Likewise, meat will test alkaline before digestion, but it leaves very acidic residue in the body, so, like nearly all animal products, meat is very acid-forming.

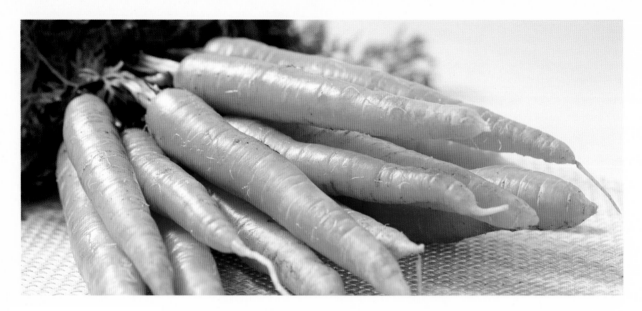

HOW ACIDIC ARE YOU?

Curious to know how balanced your body is? You can test your own acid/alkaline balance with a simple saliva test using commercial pH test strips (pHion is a good brand). The test itself is extremely easy to conduct:

1. Wait two hours after eating before taking the test.

2. When you're ready, fill your mouth with saliva and then swallow it. Repeat this step again to make sure your saliva is clean.

3. On the third time, place some of the saliva on the pH test paper.

If the paper turns blue, then you are in a healthy alkaline state at a pH of 7.4. Amazing!

If the paper does not turn blue, compare the color of your paper with the chart on the box to see how acidic you have become. Don't be discouraged by the results of your test. As I mentioned earlier, you will be able to return your body to a healthy alkaline state, and I am here to help you do just that.

SO HOW DOES A DETOX OR CLEANSE FIT IN?

Where do I even start? First, a detox helps you establish (or re-establish) a healthy relationship with food. And not just any food, the food that will help you achieve a vital life filled with boundless energy, optimal health, and unparalleled mental well-being.

It may sound difficult since you will need to give up many of your favorite foods, but the beauty of a detox is that it resets your palate and crushes your cravings so you no longer desire all those bad, acid-forming foods you used to love. And when those pesky cravings are no longer what your body is screaming for, you'll begin to notice the other messages your body is sending you, such as demands for the things it *does* need, or signs that something is amiss and needs to be addressed. You will become so in-tune with your body that you'll even be able to diagnose many health issues—which could end up saving your life one day!

Plus, once you have reset your internal environment, you'll notice the pounds start to fall off! As your blood sugar levels normalize, you'll feel fuller for longer on less food, while your body benefits from the absence of insulin spikes that used to prompt fat storage, and the increased energy that allows you to be more active.

There are many different types of detox programs, some much stricter than others. Some require you to stick to only liquids, like juices, while others allow solids in the form of raw foods, which consist of a variety of uncooked, unprocessed, unheated, and preferably organic or wild foods.

THE BENEFITS OF RAW FOODS

There are a ton of the advantages to eating raw food. First of all, dishes prepared with raw foods taste wonderful because the flavors are natural to the foods themselves. They also require fewer additives such as salt, spices, oils, and sweeteners.

Furthermore, every major health organization, medical doctor, and health and wellness practitioner recommends that we eat at least five servings of fruits and vegetables daily, preferably raw. This is because raw foods have more nutrients and fibers, since food loses a lot of its vitamin and nutrient content during the cooking process.

Raw foods are also digested more easily, usually taking 24 to 36 hours, as opposed to the 48 to 100 hours cooked food takes. This saves your body a lot of energy!

Finally, the nutrients found in raw foods strengthen the immune system, thereby preventing illness and disease. A raw diet has also been shown to improve the health of those suffering from arthritis, asthma, high blood pressure, cancer, diabetes, digestive disturbances, menstrual problems, allergies, obesity, psoriasis, skin conditions, heart disease, diverticulitis, weakened immunity, depression, and hormonal imbalances. And if that isn't enough, a raw diet causes degenerative diseases to virtually disappear. The aging process slows, the whites of your eyes will become whiter, you'll have more energy, and you'll need less sleep.

THE BENEFITS OF JUICING

Juicing has become increasingly popular over the past few years among everyone from celebrities to pro-athletes to everyday people like you and me. And for good reason: fresh juice is extremely nutrient dense and is absorbed directly into your bloodstream, where it can go to work detoxifying your body, boosting your immune system, and changing your entire internal environment for the better. On top of helping to shed unwanted pounds, studies have shown juicing improves sleep, greatly diminishes allergies, strengthens hair and nails, treats skin conditions, and even improves mental, emotional, and spiritual health. Ready to pour yourself a glass yet?

If you are, here are my top five juicing tips to help you get started!

1. Start off slowly. Your body will not be used to such a concentrated form of vitamins and minerals, so give it time to adjust. Stick to one or two juices a day for the first week or two.

2. Drink juice on an empty stomach (ideally in the morning) to allow the nutrients to pass more quickly into your intestines.

3. Juice only the best! You are looking to detoxify your body, so choose high-quality organic produce whenever possible.

4. Drink your juice immediately. As it sits, it loses many of its active ingredients. If you want to make some ahead of time, don't make more than a day or two's worth.

5. Once you've gotten the hang (and the taste) for juicing, try adding some fresh herbs.

But because you are removing the fiber, it is important to also eat whole fruits and vegetables as part of a healthy diet. Unless you are on a juice cleanse, do not get all your nutrients from juice alone.

Which leads me to . . .

THE BENEFITS OF BLENDING

One question I get asked all the time is: Which is better: juicing or blending?

In truth, both juices and smoothies can play an important role in any healthy diet, albeit in different ways. But despite the current trend toward juice cleanses, I am personally partial to blending—and here's why:

When you juice, you leave behind important fiber which is not only important for good digestion, but also helps you feel full while stabilizing blood-sugar levels.

Like juicing, blending your fruits and veggies makes them easier to digest, while still providing an amazing, nutrient-dense beverage.

Most people actually find it much easier to add tons of leafy greens to their diet when they can toss them in their blender and whizz them up with their favorite fruit and some ice. Even the simplest green smoothie can help you reap the benefits of important phytonutrients, antioxidants, and essential vitamins and minerals (think increased energy, glowing skin, and a positive mind!).

And these are just a few of the great benefits of blending!

But with all the blenders on the market, how do you choose the right one? Personally, after much trial and error, I have settled on Blendtec as my favorite. They are powerful enough to let you not only whip up gourmet caliber smoothies at home (at a fraction of the cost), but also to blend soups, homemade nut butters, and dips. Plus, they come in a variety of styles and sizes to fit in any kitchen, and there are budget-friendly options as well. And since they have a lifetime warranty, you'll be able to enjoy fresh smoothies for years and years!

FILLING YOUR PANTRY – THE RIGHT WAY

I know what you're thinking. "What do you mean? I go to the grocery store, fill my cart, pay, and leave." Well, not exactly. A hundred years ago, the way people shopped for their food was quite different. You knew your butcher (by name) and knew where his meat came from. You bought your produce directly from local farmers whose farms were mere miles away from your town, and you bought things fresh as you needed them since you didn't have the same storage capabilities we have today. Unfortunately, in our modern world, we have lost that intimate relationship we once had with our food and the people who produce it. Most of us shop at large supermarkets where you don't even know the cashier's name, let alone where all the food in your cart came from. So it is any wonder that we are feeling low, overweight, and unhealthier than ever before? Well, it doesn't have to be this way!

Try and take the way you shop back to simpler times by creating relationships with the people and places you get your food. And with that, here are my top tips for good shopping:

1. Visit local farmers markets to get your produce and hormone-free meats.

2. Buy the best quality food you can afford. And top quality doesn't have to mean top dollar. Just look for options that are as fresh and chemical- and hormone-free as possible.

3. Try and shop as you need items instead of one bulk shop. Again, the fresher your food, the better. This will also save money by not throwing away unused food!

4. Buy organic wherever possible.

5. Embrace biodynamic agriculture, a holistic approach to growing food that emphasizes the relationship between the soil, the plants, and the animals in a self-sustaining system. It is the best food for you, and the best for our planet.

6. Support organic box businesses. (If you are not familiar with these, they are services offered by local farmers whereby they deliver fresh produce right to your home.)

7. Pick small local shops that are more likely to know where their product came from. Asking questions will increase demand for more accountability when it comes to food.

8. Say no to genetically modified foods! We just don't know what they do to our bodies.

9. Skip the drive thru and the frozen food section (except frozen vegetables which can actually pack more nutrients than older fresh produce). You (and your health) are worth the small time investment to create your own wholesome, fresh meals.

10. Read the label! If you don't know how to pronounce it, you don't want it in your body. Also be sure to check the "best by" date, especially on produce.

GRASS-FED BEEF AND GAME MEAT

As we talked about earlier, red meat is very acid-forming in the body. But, I don't expect you to give up enjoying a juicy, delicious steak once in a while! However, there are ways to ensure the beef and other game meats that come across your plate are top notch, and you can do this by focusing on what *they* eat.

Not only is grass-feeding our meat better for the planet, but research shows that it is leaner and healthier for us omnivores. Why is this? For one, beef from grass-fed meat contains up to a third less fat per serving than grain-fed, and the fat it does have boasts more benefits. For example, a three-ounce serving contains 35 mg of the heart- and brain-protecting omega-3s, EPA, and DHA, compared with only 18 mg for the same serving of meat from grain-fed stock. Grass-fed beef also contains twice the conjugated linoleic acid (CLA) per serving (26 mg, compared with 13 mg in grain-fed). Higher CLA levels have been linked with easier weight loss and a reduced risk of heart disease, as well as certain types of cancer. Furthermore, grass-fed beef is substantially higher in vitamins A, E, and beta-carotene.

And a grass-munching heffer has more benefits than that! Eating grass-fed beef is less likely to make you sick, as research has reported fewer instances of E-coli in grass-fed beef than in grain-fed beef.

So where can you find it? It used to be that the best place to order your grass-fed meat would be online (and it's still an option), but now certain specialty stores, like Whole Foods, carry a variety of grass-fed cuts of meat. You should also try your local butcher shop and farmers markets, as their product is more likely to come straight from the farm, meaning they know the meat's history.

CHOOSING ORGANIC

It is true that organic has become a bit of a buzz word in the past few years, but this is not without reason. Not only do organic foods taste better, but they allow you to avoid foods laden with chemicals, known carcinogens, and artificial stimulants, while at the same time often supporting local farmers and helping the environment through a smaller carbon footprint. Furthermore, eating denatured foods that do not satisfy the body's nutritional needs leads to overeating. Is eating organic more expensive? Well, yes and no. I have found produce at my local farmers market to be a fraction of the price at the grocery store, but on the whole, organic options tend to be higher in price. If you do not have a local market and simply can't afford grocery store prices, at least avoid what I like to call the dirty dozen, which are the top most contaminated foods that you absolutely should buy organic:

» Peaches

» Apples

» Sweet Bell Peppers

» Celery

» Nectarines

» Strawberries

» Cherries

» Pears

» Grapes (Imported)

» Spinach

» Lettuce

» Potatoes

Ok . . . I know I've mentioned farmers markets numerous times now, and there may be some of you who are thinking, "What the heck is a farmers market and is there one close to me?"

Basically, a farmers market is simply a forum for local farmers to sell their products directly to consumers. They are typically open on Saturdays, and perhaps one or two days during the week, depending on the market.

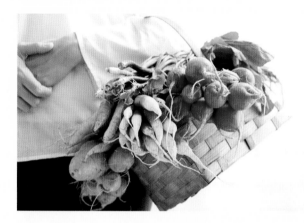

There are many reasons for choosing to shop at a local farmers market, including access to fresher and healthier seasonal foods. There is also a wider variety of wholesome choices, such as organic foods, pasture-raised meats, free-range eggs and poultry, handmade farmstead cheeses, and many less transport-immune options disfavored by large grocers. Another (big) bonus? It's cheaper! And not just a little cheaper. According to some research, up to 91% cheaper. This is most likely because the process of production is more concise, there is less distance to travel, and there are fewer middlemen.

Go online to see if there is a farmers market near you.

NO FARMERS MARKET?

That's okay. There are plenty of ways to get well on a budget, even if you don't have access to cheap, local produce. Here are some helpful tips for eating right without breaking the bank:

1. Start by checking out your local store flyers for what is on sale. Most stores post these online now, making this step super convenient!

2. Make a meal plan for the week, incorporating the items that are on sale. Try and create meals that use the same ingredients. This will save you money and cut down on waste by utilizing things like fresh herbs and produce so they don't end up in the trash at the end of the week.

3. Make a list. This is the best way to avoid impulsive buys—by having a clear outline of what you are there to purchase.

4. Don't shop hungry! It's a surefire way to end up with things you do not need, or even want, since almost everything looks tasty on an empty stomach.

5. Prepare your own meals whenever possible. We all know that dining out is expensive, but it also gives you less control over the food you're eating. Save it for special occasions or for a treat every now and then.

6. Plan for leftovers! I always try and make a little extra at dinner time to make lunch the next day a snap, saving both time *and* money.

7. Choose smaller portions. Eating less is not only good for your waistline, but it's good for your wallet too!

8. Avoid pre-packaged snacks. They are not only often the unhealthiest, but you pay a premium

for those individual-sized packages! Make your own ready-to-go baggies of snacks, such as unsalted and raw nuts, apples, or veggie sticks and keep them on hand for when you need a quick bite on-the-go.

9. Grow your own. Buying fresh herbs to add a nice kick to your meals can get expensive, especially when you're usually throwing them out every week! Growing your own herbs indoors or outdoors is easy and economical. Most stores sell popular herb plants like basil, rosemary, and thyme. Just pop them on your windowsill or plant them in a planter and enjoy fresh herbs whenever you like!

10. Buy in bulk. Items such as grains, certain vegetables such as baby carrots, and even meat are often cheaper when bought in bulk. Grains last a long time in your cupboard, and meat is easily frozen, so take advantage of the savings.

HOW TO PREPARE YOUR FOOD AND EAT IT TOO!

Bringing awareness to how you prepare and eat your food can bring a sense of enjoyment and mindfulness that you didn't know was possible with such simple acts. And this newfound pleasure is bound to change your relationship with food, making maintaining healthy eating habits that much easier.

When it comes to preparing your food, the best ways are often the simplest. Starting with fresh ingredients that are thoroughly washed is a must. For produce, discard any bad parts or outer leaves that are damaged, and begin cutting and slicing when you are ready to cook so as to preserve as many nutrients as possible. I am a fan of pre-prep where possible, because I understand the time constraints

of a busy schedule. But when you do have the time (and try and make it where you can), don't pre-cut fruits and vegetables.

When you are ready to start cooking, bring your full attention to what you are doing. Think about where your food came from, who grew it, and be grateful for its presence and all the goodness it will provide you and your body. In some Indian cultures, it is customary to chant or meditate while cooking so your food can absorb all the positive energy you

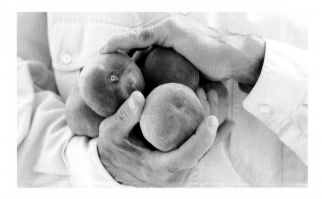

are channeling. This might not be your kitchen style, but a little love added to any recipe is never a bad addition to a meal! So get those positive vibes flowing.

Once you have sat down to enjoy the meal you prepared, shift your awareness to eating it. Many of us rush through our meals in front of the TV, answering emails, or even walking down the street on our way to a meeting, but as much focus should be paid to enjoying a meal as is paid to making it. Food should be eaten slowly, with intent, and at a proper table. Here are some tips for achieving mindful eating:

» Mind your posture when sitting at the table, keeping your back as straight as you comfortably can. Also, some fresh flowers or a soft glowing candle enhances the experience.

» Turn off the television, shut down your computer, and switch off your cell phone. Bring your full attention to your food and enjoying it. But good conversation is more than okay!

» You took the time to prepare the food, so take some time to present it properly on your plate. A little pride in your work is necessary.

» Take in your food with your other senses before tasting it.

» Practice some deep breathing. Not only does this act help your body become more alkaline, but it helps you bring awareness to your meal.

» When you take a bite, take the time to savor it. Notice not only its taste, but its texture, its temperature, and its complexity.

» Chew! Many of us wolf down food like we're in famine, but chewing is an important step in allowing the digestive enzymes in our saliva to begin to break down food and start the digestive process. Aim to chew 8 to 12 times before swallowing.

» Warm herbal teas and room temperature water with your meal is an excellent way to aid digestion so you get the most out of your food.

» Slow down by putting your fork and knife down between each bite. This will allow you to notice when you start to feel full, signaling that it's time to stop eating. Unlike when you were a child, no one is forcing you to finish your plate!

HERBS—NATURE'S HEALERS

For thousands of years, ancient civilizations harnessed the power of certain herbs for their medicinal and healing qualities. In fact, most modern medicines actually originated from herbs. For example, Aspirin-salicin was actually first found in the White Willow herb. Digitalin, a group of medicines used today for heart conditions, are extracted from foxglove plants.

When taken properly, herbs can be an amazingly effective way to support your body's natural detox processes, while also bestowing upon you their healing and restorative properties. They can also help combat some of the symptoms you will experience when cleansing. Since the toxins you are releasing from your body have been settled in your cells and organs for some time, they can create some discomfort when they re-enter your bloodstream on their way out of your body. Incorporating herbs into your detox will help soothe symptoms such as headaches, fatigue, nausea, and insomnia.

Here are some of the best "powerhouse" herbs and their benefits. Try adding them to your salads, soup, juices, and sauces to take advantage of their amazing healing qualities.

Basil—*helps treat depression and anxiety while also boasting antiseptic and anti-nausea properties. It even helps soothe coughs!*

Chamomile—*has anti-inflammatory and anti-nausea properties. It also has calming effects that can greatly aid sleep, reduce stress, and treat anxiety. It can also help those suffering from IBS and indigestion. Works best when brewed as a tea.*

Dandelion—*helps detox the kidneys, liver, and digestive tract. It is also a powerful diuretic, anti-rheumatic, and anti-toxin.*

Fennel—*this licorice-flavored treat is a breath freshener and appetite suppressant, while also good for soothing coughs and sore throats. It is also great at relieving indigestion.*

Lemon Balm—*acts to relax and soothe while also boasting anti-depressant properties. It aids digestion by relaxing peripheral blood vessels and has antiviral and anti-bacterial qualities.*

Mint—*helps with flatulence, indigestion, travel sickness, and even soothes migraines (works best as an oil rubbed on your temples).*

Rosemary—*fragrant and delicious, it improves circulation, encourages proper digestion, boosts energy, and even soothes headaches. It's also good to have around during a cold since it treats chills and rheumatism.*

Sage—*this memory-enhancing herb is an amazing liver stimulant. It also improves digestion and circulation, and has been shown to decrease the symptoms of menopause. It also has antiseptic properties.*

Thyme—*while great for flavoring pork, this herb also improves digestion, soothes diarrhea, stomach troubles, and can effectively treat IBS.*

One of the easiest (and most relaxing) ways to enjoy herbs is in a hot, soothing cup of tea. Below are some of what I believe are the best cleansing herbal teas that can have amazing benefits to your overall wellness, both mentally and physically.

GINGER AND LEMON HERBAL TEA

As discussed earlier, ginger has amazing healing and weight loss–aiding properties. And when it comes together with lemon, a beautiful detoxifying relationship is born! Ginger has been used for thousands of years by many civilizations in folk

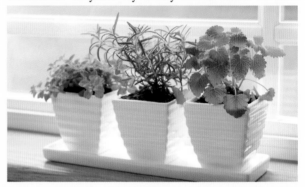

medicine, with many societies believing ginger to be healing for the liver. Lemons contain vitamin C, a powerful antioxidant that research has shown to have cell reparative properties while also blocking damage from free radicals (oxidizing agents that attack the body), including in the liver, which is quite possibly the most important organ for detoxifying your body!

GREEN TEA

Green tea is one of the most commonly used teas in the world. Not only has it been shown to support weight loss efforts by increasing metabolism, research has found that the chemicals in green tea also boost detox enzymes in the human body. And like ginger and lemon tea, it is loaded with antioxidants. Another bonus? Because it's so popular, it's readily available pretty much anywhere.

FENUGREEK AND HIBISCUS TEA

A unique mixture historically drank by the ancient Egyptians as a detox tonic, fenugreek and hibiscus tea is believed to have many detoxifying properties. First, it has been found to work as a natural laxative, cleaning out the digestive system. It has also been found to lower levels of harmful cholesterol through hibiscus's cholesterol-lowering properties. Fenugreek has also been shown to lower blood glucose levels in people with Type 2 diabetes, as well as improving problems associated with high blood glucose, such as insulin resistance.

LICORICE TEA

Licorice, or Glycyrrhiza glabra, derives its name from the Greek "glyks," meaning sweet and "rhiza," meaning root. The ancient Greeks, Romans, and Chinese were the first to use it medicinally, distilling the root and prescribing it for a wide variety of health conditions. Today it is used primarily to treat digestive and inflammation disorders, but it has also been shown to soothe kidney and bowel irritations, strengthen the liver, cleanse the colon, and provide a mild laxative effect, making it an excellent addition to any detox program. In addition to all that, licorice is also known as the "sweet root," with a delicious flavor that is actually 50 times sweeter than sugar. And at zero calories, it's the perfect treat to stave off those sugar cravings!

Other teas that will support your cleanse are:

Digestion Aid:

Meadowsweet flowers/leaf, Peppermint, Fennel seed, Marshmallow, Ginger

Super Cleansing:

Burdock, Red Clover, Alfalfa, Pau dArco, Dandelion Leaf, Cleavers, Oregon Grape

Stress Busting:

Eleuthero, Schizandra, Reishi, Ashwagandha, Holy Basil, Fo-ti, Sarsaparilla, Licorice

Energy Boosting (great for coffee drinkers!):

Ramon Nut, Yerba Mate (ground), Raw Cacao, Sarsaparilla, Maca, Roasted Dandelion

You can make almost any dried herb into an herbal tea. Start by pouring boiling water over the loose herb (1 part herb to 10 parts water) and allow it to steep for about 4 hours. When done steeping, strain it and reheat it gently before enjoying. Try it iced if you are cleansing in a hot climate or in the summer months.

HOW TO SOURCE YOUR HERBS

Whenever possible, find a supplier that purchases or grows plant medicines that are either certified organic, grown without chemicals if sourcing from small scale farmers, or wild crafted (collected in the wild).

HOW TO STORE YOUR HERBS

Three main factors affect the life of dried herbs: heat, light, and oxygen. To keep herbs at their best, store them in an air-tight container in a cool, dry place away from the light.

HOW LONG DO THEY LAST?

Dried herbs generally have a shelf life of 2 years. Alcohol extracts or tinctures have a longer shelf life of 15–20 years, because they are preserved in alcohol.

Remember, when it comes to herbs too much of a good thing can be a bad thing. Make sure you talk to your health care professional before beginning any herbal regimen.

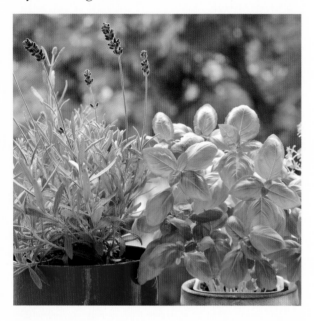

SUPERFOODS – SUPER HEALTH!

These nutrient-dense foods are the superstars of any healthy diet and should be consumed often. Packed with vitamins, minerals, and so many other amazing nutrients, these foods need to become part of your regular mealtime rotation!

SALMON

Salmon offers the dynamic duo of fat burning: protein and fish oil. You might already know that protein does a great job of revving the metabolism. But what you might not know is what fish oil can do. According to numerous research studies, the right amount of the kind of omega-3 fats found in fish oil can boost metabolism by a whopping 400 calories each day. And it does this while fighting diabetes, heart disease, and cancer.

OMEGA-3 EGGS

Omega-3 eggs also pack a one-two, protein- omega-3 punch. Protein combined with the heart-healthy, disease-fighting, metabolism-boosting omega-3 fats is a hard combo to beat. And don't fear the yolk: that's where the omega-3s are.

LOW-FAT PLAIN GREEK YOGURT

Greek yogurt is a smooth and creamy way to boost the protein and calcium content of your diet. Research from the University of Tennessee shows that increased calcium intake speeds the metabolism and promotes fat loss.

SPINACH

Spinach ranks #1 on the veggie list because of its strong base content. A spinach salad or some cooked spinach can neutralize nearly any dietary acid-forming food, and that's good for both bones and muscles. Spinach is also high in fiber, which improves gastrointestinal health and promotes fat loss. It's also got folic acid for reducing the risk of heart disease, cancer, and memory loss associated with aging.

TOMATOES

In addition to tasting delicious and offering a good dose of fiber and vitamin C, cooked tomatoes (even those in tomato sauce) are rich in lycopene. An increase in lycopene intake can result in a 50% reduction in the risk of heart disease and prostate cancer.

CRUCIFEROUS VEGETABLES (BROCCOLI, CABBAGE, CAULIFLOWER)

These vegetables contain a special class of nutrients called indoles that have been found to protect against a variety of cancers, balance hormones, and offer antioxidant benefits. They are also high in fiber.

AVOCADOS

Avocados are probably the healthiest fruits on the block. They contain a heaping portion of B-vitamins, fiber, folic acid, and zinc (among other nutrients). They also provide a healthy dose of monounsaturated fats.

MIXED BERRIES (STRAWBERRIES, BLUEBERRIES, RASPBERRIES, ETC.)

Berries are one of the best antioxidant foods around. In fact, they rank highest in their ability to soak up cell-damaging oxygen free radicals. These tiny fruits also have amazing anti-aging properties.

ORANGES

Oranges are best known for their vitamin C content. But they also happen to be great sources of fiber and folic acid.

QUINOA (ANCIENT GRAINS)

The nutritive properties of quinoa have given it the title of super grain. This is largely due to the fact that quinoa is rich in a variety of energy-producing vitamins and minerals such as calcium, magnesium, iron, phosphorous, and B-vitamins. In addition to these benefits, quinoa is one of the only grains that provide complete protein. Finally, because quinoa contains no gluten, it's the best grain for those with gastrointestinal problems associated with other grains.

MIXED NUTS (PECANS, WALNUTS, CASHEWS, BRAZIL NUTS, ETC.)

While nuts used to be considered bad news because of the fat, we now know nuts are one of the healthiest foods around. Eating nuts regularly has been shown to decrease the risks for several diseases (including heart disease), and to promote weight loss. This is due to the fact that nuts are rich in dietary fiber, magnesium, copper, folic acid, potassium, and vitamin E. In addition, they're loaded with healthy polyunsaturated and monounsaturated fats that speed up metabolism.

STEEL CUT OATS

Oats and quinoa run neck and neck for the title of healthiest grain, so both should be included in a healthy diet. Oats have a low glycemic index and therefore greatly help in controlling blood sugars. They are also rich in the B-vitamins and vitamin E, are more hypo allergenic when compared to wheat and other grains, and contain more soluble fiber than any other grain.

EXTRA-VIRGIN OLIVE OIL

It should come as no surprise that this cornerstone of the Mediterranean diet is on our healthy foods list. The monounsaturated fats that come from olive oil play a role in reducing the risk for a variety of diseases, and to increase the metabolism.

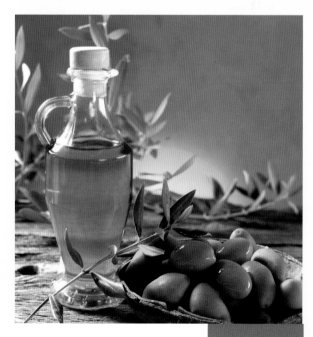

FISH OIL (SALMON, ANCHOVY, MENHADEN)

The specific fats (EPA and DHA) in fish oils are considered to be a cure-all by some experts. Fish oil supplementation has been shown to reduce depression, protect against virtually every disease in modern society, boost muscle mass, reduce body fat, and speed up metabolism. Taking 6 to 10 grams of fish oil (via supplements) per day is the best way to fast track your way to all of these benefits.

SPIRULINA

Spirulina is a type of blue-green algae that is rich in protein, vitamins, minerals, and carotenoids, antioxidants that can help protect cells from damage. It contains nutrients like B-vitamins, beta-carotene, vitamin E, manganese, zinc, copper, iron, selenium, and gamma linolenic acid (an essential fatty acid). It also supports the immune system, helps rebuild blood cells, improves gastrointestinal health, and balances the microflora in the gut. However, like any blue-green algae, it can be contaminated with toxic substances called microcystins and can also absorb heavy metals from the water where it is grown, so make sure to buy spirulina from a trusted brand.

BEE POLLEN

Bee pollen is the food of young bees, and it is approximately 40% protein. It is considered one of nature's most completely nourishing foods because it contains nearly all nutrients required by humans. About half of its protein is in the form of free amino acids that are ready to be used immediately by the body. It is also reported that bee pollen in the diet acts to normalize cholesterol and triglyceride levels in the blood, and works wonders in a weight-control or weight-stabilization regimen by correcting a possible chemical imbalance in body metabolism that may be involved in either abnormal weight gain or loss.

BREWER'S YEAST

Brewer's yeast comes from the dried-up cells of the Saccharomyces cerevisiae fungus, a one-celled organism used to brew beer. This long-used nutritional supplement comes in powder, flake, liquid and tablet forms, and contains healthy amounts of the B-complex vitamins, chromium, and protein. The protein and chromium found in brewer's yeast can help you lose unwanted pounds or maintain a healthy weight by reducing your levels of body fat. Brewer's yeast is also a rich source of various B-vitamins, which can help to alleviate symptoms of depression, particularly irritability and nervousness, as well as reduce signs of aging. It can also help you treat certain skin conditions such as acne flare-ups, and eczema, and can help strengthen brittle nails and dry hair.

MACA ROOT POWDER

Maca is a nutritionally dense super-food that contains high amounts of minerals, vitamins, enzymes, and all of the essential amino acids. Maca root is rich in B-vitamins, the "energy vitamins," and is a vegetarian source of vitamin B12. In addition, maca has high levels of bioavailable calcium and magnesium and is great for remineralization. Another fantastic benefit is it helps balance our hormones, which tend to be out of whack due to an over abundance of environmental estrogens and lifestyle choices. And because it stimulates the hypothalamus and pituitary glands, which regulate the other glands, maca also balances the adrenal, thyroid, pancreas, ovarian, and testicular glands. Maca root has also been shown to be beneficial for treating PMS, menopause, and hot flashes, and can also enhance fertility.

MATCHA GREEN TEA

Matcha green tea has been consumed for hundreds of years by Buddhist monks, samurai warriors, and millions of Japanese because of all the amazing health benefits it provides simply by drinking it once per day. The green tea leaf is world renowned for its weight loss benefits, antioxidant content, energy boosting properties, and so much more. Studies show that matcha green tea extract has unique thermogenic properties that promote increased fat oxidation and increases thermogenesis (the rate your body burns calories) from 10% to 40% of daily energy use. In other words, matcha green tea increases your body's ability to burn fat and calories by 4 times. It has also been shown that drinking a cup of matcha green tea before physical activity can result in a 25% increase in fat burning during the activity. Furthermore, despite having less caffeine than coffee, green tea gives you clean boost of energy that can last up to 6 hours. It is also rich in L-Theanine, a rare amino acid that affects the brain's functioning to promote a state of well-being, alertness, and relaxation.

SPROUTING

Spouted seeds and grains are some of the most nutrient dense, enzymatically-active, alkalizing foods you can eat. You may be familiar with alfalfa and broccoli sprouts, but today there is a plethora of varieties available, including quinoa, red clover, radish, mung beans, fenugreek, chickpeas, and lentils. And growing them in your home is easy! All you need are three readily available household objects: a jar, cheesecloth (or fine mesh), and a rubber band. Here are the ten steps for sprouting:

1. Rinse the seeds you intend to sprout well and pour into the jar (fill to ¼ mark).

2. Fill the jar at least ¾ full of water.

3. Soak overnight at room temperature.

4. Pour out the water and seeds and rinse with fresh water.

5. Return the seeds to the jar.

6. Cover the jar with cheesecloth or mesh and secure with the rubber band.

7. Briefly turn the jar upside down to drain the remaining water.

8. Sprouts will begin to appear within 24 hours (give or take).

9. Make sure the sprouts stay moist so they sprout fully by rinsing and draining them and keep them warm and away from direct sunlight (so no windowsills).

10. As they sprout, pick and enjoy! But make sure to rinse your sprouts before eating.

11. Sprouts can be stored in the fridge uncovered for up to one week.

Toss them in your salads or munch them as they are—just get them into your diet! However, it should be noted that some people may have an allergy to sprouts, so if you're new to sprouting, be aware of any allergic symptoms.

WHEATGRASS

Wheatgrass is another superfood I can't promote enough. It detoxifies, cleanses the colon, purifies the blood, and has a vast array of cancer-fighting properties. It is also high in vitamin K, B6, calcium, and is a great source of protein. However, because it is very detoxifying, some may experience nausea when they first start drinking it. This is because it starts an immediate reaction with the toxins and the mucus in the stomach. Therefore, I recommend that beginners start with 1 ounce of juiced wheatgrass a day mixed with water, and then slowly work more into your diet (up to 6 ounces per day).

Wheatgrass can be hard to come by if you don't have a juice bar or organic store nearby. But like sprouts, growing your own is simple. Here's how:

1. Buy the seeds at a local organic store or online.

2. Fill a seed tray with 1 inch of general compost.

3. Add the seeds to the compost and water.

4. Water daily and keep them in a warm place away from direct sunlight.

5. Your wheatgrass should be grown and ready to cut in 6 days. Continue to plant and grow in order to keep yourself stocked with a ready supply.

MILK AND DAIRY

Aside from organic, plain yogurt (preferably Greek or goat for the high protein content), I am not a proponent of including dairy in your diet. Here is why:

Dairy products are very acid-forming and have been linked to a host of health problems, including acne, anemia, anxiety, arthritis, attention deficit disorder, attention deficit hyperactivity disorder, fibromyalgia, headaches, heartburn, indigestion, irritable bowel syndrome, joint pain, osteoporosis, poor immune function, allergies, ear infections, colic, obesity, heart disease, diabetes, autism, Crohn's disease, breast and prostate cancers, and ovarian cancer.

Furthermore, mammals need the enzyme lactase to digest lactose (the sugar bond in dairy). However, between the ages of 18 months and 4 years, we lose 90 to 95 percent of this enzyme. The undigested lactose and the acidic nature of pasteurized milk encourages the growth of bacteria in our intestines.

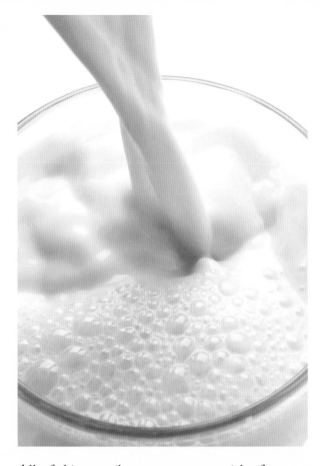

All of this contributes to a greater risk of cancer, because cancer cells thrive in acidic conditions. In addition, dairy products produce mucus, and often the body will develop a cold or allergies to fight the dairy invasion.

Instead, I recommend the following as great substitutes:

» Organic, unsweetened homemade almond milk

» Organic, unsweetened homemade hemp milk

» Kefir

Some nutritionists include soy milk on their list of alternatives, but I do not. Soy isoflavones are classified as endocrine disruptors, and have the potential to cause negative effects on reproductive health, fertility, infant development, and even brain development. So unless you are a woman who is low in estrogen, I recommend that you steer clear.

ROUNDING OUT NUTRITION WITH SUPPLEMENTS

Even with a healthy, balanced diet it can still be difficult to get the Recommended Daily Allowance (RDA) of vitamins and minerals from our food alone. That's why I recommend introducing a high-quality multivitamin and specific supplements into your diet, guaranteeing you get all the nutrients your body needs. Below is my list of the top vitamins and supplements needed for achieving optimal health:

ACES Blend Multivitamin—this blend combines four important vitamins and minerals: vitamins A, C, E, and Selenmium. Vitamin A is a fat soluble vitamin that is stored in our liver. It contributes to normal growth and development while keeping our eyes, skin, and immune system healthy. The famous vitamin C helps protect against immune system deficiencies, cardiovascular disease, prenatal health problems, eye disease, and even skin wrinkling. Vitamin E is used for many purposes, mainly for treating and preventing diseases of the heart and blood vessels, including hardening of the arteries, heart attack, chest pain, leg pain due to blocked arteries, and high blood pressure. It is also used for treating diabetes and its complications, and has been shown to play a role in preventing cancer, particularly lung and oral cancer in smokers; colorectal cancer and polyps; and gastric, prostate, and pancreatic

cancer. Lastly, Selenium, a mineral found in the soil, has been shown to protect cells from free-radical damage, enable your thyroid to produce thyroid hormone (thus affecting weight loss), and help lower your risk of joint inflammation. Throw all of these together and that is one powerful vitamin cocktail!

Omega-3—as discussed earlier, oily fish such as salmon, trout, and herring are excellent sources of omega-3 fatty acids, which are associated with protective effects on the heart and so many other amazing health benefits. Luckily, you can get all of these benefits from a bottle by taking a fish oil supplement. 600 to 1000 mg per day is the typical recommended dosage.

Vitamin D—most people associate vitamin D with the sun and the blues that accompany a deficiency of it. But vitamin D is also responsible for helping your body absorb calcium, working together to help you maintain healthy bones and teeth. It also helps your muscles, nerves, and immune system work properly. Recent research has shown that vitamin D may be linked to lowering the risk of diseases such as multiple sclerosis and some cancers. Most people should aim to get approximately 600 IU (international units) per day.

Glutamine—glutamine is the most abundant free amino acid (the building blocks of protein) in the body. It is produced in the muscles and is distributed by the blood to the organs that need it. Glutamine has been shown to help gut function, the immune system, and other essential processes in the body, especially in times of stress. It is also important for providing "fuel" (nitrogen and carbon) to many different cells in the body. Lastly, glutamine is needed to make other chemicals in the body, such as other amino acids and glucose (sugar). The most common supplement form is 500 mg capsules.

Zinc—this essential trace element is needed for the proper growth and maintenance of the human body. It is found in several systems and biological reactions, and it is needed for immune function, wound healing, blood clotting, thyroid function, and much more. Zinc is responsible for boosting the immune system, treating the common cold and recurrent ear infections, and preventing lower respiratory infections. It has also been used to treat certain eye conditions, such as macular degeneration, night blindness, and cataracts. It is also used for asthma, diabetes, high blood pressure, acquired immunodeficiency syndrome (AIDS), and skin conditions such as psoriasis, eczema, and acne.

Plant-based and whey protein—whey protein is derived from whey, which is a by-product of cheese produced from cow's milk. Of all the protein sources, it provides the highest amount of branch-chained amino acids (BCAAs), which aid with muscle growth and retention. It is also absorbed by the body with spectacular speed and has been shown to have positive benefits for the immune system. Hemp and soy proteins are excellent vegetarian sources of protein. Both contain all 21 amino acids. However, both have their weaknesses. Soy is said to be the second most allergenic food to humans, and is also known to cause slight raises in the body's estrogen levels. Unlike soy, allergies toward hemp protein are virtually nonexistent, but hemp protein tends to be higher in fat. No matter which one you choose, the great news is all of these proteins are available in powder form, perfect for adding to your favorite smoothie for a morning protein boost!

Chia, flax, and hemp seeds/oil—despite being prized by the ancient Aztecs, chia just recently became a sort of celebrity in the nutrition world as the new superfood. This is because 1 tablespoon of these little guys packs 2 grams of protein, 4 grams of fiber, and 1.75 grams omega-3s! Offering a similar nutritional punch, 1 Tbsp. of flax seeds boasts 2 grams of protein, 3 grams of fiber, 13% daily value of manganese, and 2 grams omega-3s. They also deliver more ALA (Alpha-Linolenic Acid, an essential fatty acid that cannot be produced by the body) than any other plant food. But make sure you grind them up (you can use a coffee grinder) before adding them to food, since their outer shell prevents your body from digesting the seeds. Then we have hemp seeds. Just 1 tablespoon packs 4 grams of protein, 16% daily value of phosphorus, 16% daily value of magnesium, and 1 gram of omega-3s. Try sprinkling a tablespoon of any one of these amazing seeds onto a salad, into a shake or smoothie, or on top of a morning bowl of oatmeal!

Coconut Butter—this delicious treat made from the meat of the coconut has many awesome health benefits. First of all, it has been shown to boost immunity, kill bacteria and viruses, protect against cancer and other degenerative diseases, and prevent osteoporosis by promoting calcium absorption. It may also slow down aging and is good for skin radiance! Although it is technically a saturated fat, unlike animal fats, coconut butter contains healthy, healing, medium chain triglycerides (MCTs). This saturated fat is considered a rare and important building block of every cell in the human body, and can actually reduce cholesterol and heart disease. Substitute it into your favorite recipes to enjoy all the health benefits it has to offer.

It is important to make sure you use supplements from reputable brands. I recommend the following supplement brands: *Sun Warrior, Manitoba Harvest, Precision, Natural Factors, Sisu, Progressive, New Chapter, Genuine Health, Vega, Ascenta Nutrasea, Allmax, Dymatize, Udo's, Genestra, Flora Smart, Floradix,* and *NOW.*

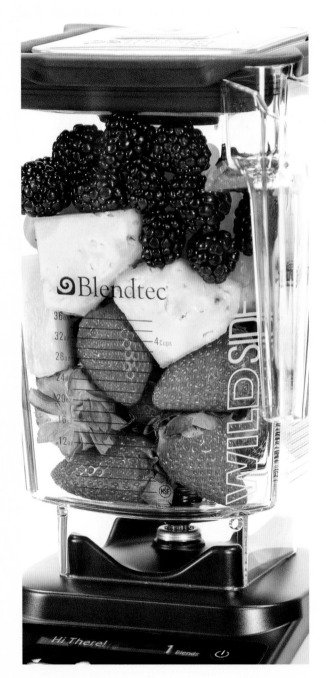

As I mentioned earlier, detox programs are fun and easy, as long as you start with the right attitude and the right prep! Here are some things you can do to help you get started, stay organized, and ensure your success.

GET THE RIGHT TOOLS

TOOLS FOR THE KITCHEN

Just like you can't clean your home without a few supplies, the same is true for your body! Over the next 21 days, you will need access to a few things to create the meals in the recipe section included in this book, as well as to stay organized, which will make sticking to the program that much easier. Below is a list of items you will need to pick up in order to get started:

» A blender or juicer

» A sharp knife

» A cutting board

» A water bottle

» Plastic containers to store soups and juices (most recipes make 2–3 servings at least)

» A journal to track your moods, food, and progress

TOOLS FOR GETTING MOVING

Fitness is an important component in achieving optimal health. It reduces the risk of disease, improves your energy and stamina, burns fat and tones your body, and improves your mood by releasing powerful endorphins. It's true that when cleansing, you want to give your body lots of rest and the ability to use its energy to expel all those toxins. But there are some great low-impact activities you can partake in that will benefit you greatly while encouraging the cleansing process. Therefore, you will need a few basic things:

» Comfortable workout attire

» Proper running shoes

» Sports bag

Depending on what type of activity you choose, you may also need:

» Yoga mat

» Light hand-held weights

» Bicycle

PLAN AHEAD

In today's busy world, the biggest saboteur of a healthy lifestyle is lack of time. It's the perfect excuse for bailing on your evening workout, for grabbing that burger at the drive thru, or for skipping a meal altogether. Being prepared and planning ahead is the most important component of successfully maintaining any new nutrition plan. Not only does it bust the excuses, but it also makes your life much easier, and who doesn't want that?

One of the best ways to save time in the kitchen is by prepping your fruits and veggies ahead of time. I like to wash, slice, and store a few days worth of salad ingredients, as well as dressings, so throwing together a healthy meal is effortless. Also, having a container of peeled and frozen bananas in the freezer for smoothies is not only a big help, but

freezing the bananas helps break down the starches, making them easier to digest.

When you do have time, try and prepare and eat your meals within the same 24 hours as this ensures you get the maximum nutritional value. Smoothies and juices can be stored in the fridge for up to 24 hours in an airtight sealed glass jar. It is totally okay to make your juices for the following day the night before to cut down on the morning rush.

Life is hectic, but planning ahead will ensure that you reach your goals no matter what it throws your way!

ADAPTING MEAL PLANS

Although it is my intention that you stick as close to the meal plans I have designed as possible, it is okay to make substitutions if you have allergies or just really don't like a certain food. Of course, I encourage you to give fruits, vegetables, or herbs that you don't like another try before giving up on them entirely. Sometimes our taste buds actually change when you begin to eat new foods on a regular basis, so be open to letting your tongue make those adjustments! If you absolutely cannot stomach the flavor of a certain ingredient, leave it out or find a substitute you enjoy.

ACCOUNTABILITY AND SUPPORT

For most people trying to create lasting change, having the proper support can mean the difference between success and failure. Sharing your goals and intentions with your family and friends is a great way to include them in your journey and garner their support along the way. Also, there are countless support groups, both online and offline, where you can talk with other people working toward the same goal. You can share ideas, inspirational stories, and tips for staying motivated. So make an effort to reach out. After all, we all need a little help sometimes! I will be hosting a Facebook forum where you can connect with the other participants of this program, an excellent resource I encourage you to take advantage of. Another great tool is smartphone apps, most of which not only let you interact with others who are on a similar journey as yours, but also act as a digital food diary and calorie tracker.

But going beyond simply getting the necessary support needed to succeed, sharing your journey with others also holds you accountable for the choices you make along the way—both good and bad. Being accountable to both yourself and others is an important component of successfully reaching your goals. You are far less likely to cheat on your meal plan or skip your workout when it means being honest about it to someone else. How accountable have you been to others and to yourself in the past? Are there actions you can take that would make yourself more accountable during this program? Remember, it's not about feeling guilty for the failures. It's about sharing the successes! If you haven't already enlisted the support of family, friends, or other people with similar goals as yours, do so today.

EATING OUT

Most of us suffer from the time crunch that accompanies our busy lives, and because of this I know it won't always be possible to follow the meal plan in this program 100% of the time (although it is important to make the best effort to follow it as much as possible).

When the situation arises where you need to eat out due to social obligations, travel, or work, there are a few ways you can ensure that you stick with the whole, clean foods involved in this program.

SKIP THE "NAUGHTIES"

Avoid any food that is fried, breaded, processed, and full of fat, sugar, chemicals, and other ingredients avoided during this cleanse (and hopefully for the rest of your new, healthy life). Instead, opt for a fresh salad with lemon squeezed over it as a dressing.

DO SOME RESEARCH

Lots of restaurants post their nutritional information online, allowing you to research the healthiest options available. But keep portion sizes in mind. Many places provide nutritional info for smaller servings than they actually serve you, so be mindful. Due to increased demand, here are also lots of vegetarian, vegan, and raw cafes you can try. However, these places are often trying to create unique dishes that you would not create at home, and they can still be high fat. Again, be mindful of your choices and continue to enjoy your fresh, home cooked meals whenever possible.

Visit this link for a list of many popular restaurants national info:

http://www.sparkpeople.com/resource/sparkdining.asp

SWEET TREATS

Much like the raw, vegan, and vegetarian movement is increasing the demand for eateries that cater to this lifestyle, there is also an increase in organic bakeries that offer a plethora of sweet treats. It's okay to experiment and indulge in a treat here and there. Just remember, if your goal is to shed excess weight during the next 21 days, raw and organic desserts should be eaten minimally and not used as a crutch.

ASK POLITELY

Almost all restaurants are able to accommodate special meal requests, but you need to know what to ask for. For example, ask for a large green salad, without any cheeses, meats, or high-fat toppings (like candied nuts), with an avocado to add creaminess. You can also request balsamic vinegar if you need more of a dressing. Other great restaurant meal swaps are a large plate of steamed vegetables without oil and salt, using lettuce or a bed of greens instead of a bun, bowls of fresh fruit, and vegetable-based soups.

EAT BEFORE

It's an obvious truth that when you are hungry, you are more likely to give in to temptation. Help stave off those weak moments by eating before you go out. Have a large salad, a fresh vegetable juice, or a handful of nuts or seeds to fill up and increase your chances of steering clear of bad food choices while out and about. This also works well before a dinner out at a restaurant.

BE PREPARED

You can often avoid eating out on-the-go altogether by keeping snacks readily available. Apples, cut-up vegetables, protein shakes or juices, raw and unsalted nuts, and organic protein bars make excellent options when you are out and about and need a quick snack. Simply toss them in your purse or car and you're set!

INITIATE A DAILY RITUAL

The single most important thing you can do every day to effortlessly release weight (and keep it off), boost mood, balance hormones, and support proper detoxification is to engage in daily "renewal rituals."

Renewal rituals are activities that allow the body to release the negative energy and emotions that build up in your body's tissues due to stress. These are the emotions that leave you feeling depressed, anxious, craving sweets or junk, and holding onto fat. If you don't release these negative energies and stress build-ups, then your body will intuitively find another way to cope, and often that means seeking comfort from food (especially sugar and carbs), alcohol, cigarettes, or other drugs.

A renewal ritual is something that connects you to your breath, body, and soul. In holistic medicine, it's understood that when you connect to the soul or spirit, you release positive endorphins and reduce stress hormones. And excess stress hormones are what make your body hold onto fat and age more quickly.

I recommend taking part in a renewal ritual at least once per day (ideally twice per day—morning and before dinner) since the endorphin boost lasts for only about 8 hours.

HERE ARE A FEW RITUALS you can incorporate into your daily routine over the next 21 days:

THE SUN SALUTATION

This is one of the most well-known and easily performed yoga routines you can practice in your own home. Historically, this series of poses was performed by ancient Indian monks facing the rising sun, paying homage to the sun god of health and longevity.

There are thirteen postures in total. At first you may seem off balance, uncoordinated, and awkward, but stick with it! As you practice, your movements will become more fluid, allowing you to move smoothly from one pose to the next. Start with just one complete repetition of all thirteen movements, then slowly work your way up to twelve repetitions.

Here are the instructions for The Sun Salutation routine:

1. **Namaskar** (salute)—Start in a standing position, facing the sun. Both your feet should touch each other, palms joined together, in prayer pose.

2. **Ardha Chandrasana** (Half Moon Pose)—With a deep inhalation, raise both arms above your head and tilt slightly backward arching your back.

3. **Padangusthasana** (Hand to Foot Pose)—With a deep exhalation, bend forward and touch the mat, both palms in line with your feet, forehead touching your knees.

4. **Surya Darshan** (Sun Sight Pose)—With a deep inhalation, take your right leg away from your body, in a big backward step. Both your hands should be firmly planted on your mat, your left foot between your hands, head tilted toward the ceiling.

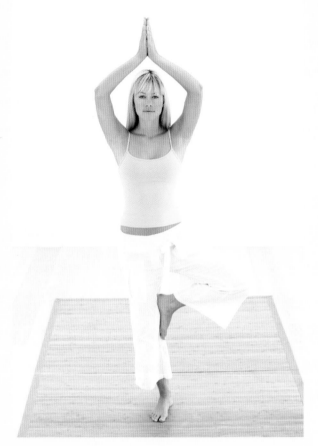

5. **Purvottanasana** (Inclined Plane)—As you breathe in, take the left leg back and bring the whole body in a straight line.

6. **Adho Mukha Svanasana** (Downward Facing Dog Pose)—With a deep exhalation, shove your hips and butt up toward the ceiling, forming an upward arch. Your arms should be straight and aligned with your head.

7. **Sashtang Dandawat** (Forehead, Chest, Knee to Floor Pose)—With a deep exhalation, lower your body down till your forehead, chest, knees, hands and feet are touching the mat, your butt tilted up. Take a normal breath in this pose.

8. **Bhujangasana** (Cobra Pose)—With a deep inhalation, slowly snake forward till your head is up, and your back is arched concave as much as possible.

9. **Adho Mukha Svanasana** (Downward Facing Dog Pose)—Exhaling deeply, again push your butt and hips up toward the ceiling as in position 6, arms aligned straight with your head.

10. **Surya Darshan** (Sun Sight Pose)—Inhaling deeply, bring your right foot in toward your body, in a big forward step. Both your hands should planted firmly on your mat, right foot between your hands, head tilted toward the ceiling.

11. **Padangusthasana** (Hand to Foot Pose)—Exhaling deeply, rise up and touch the mat, keeping both your palms in line with your feet, forehead touching your knees.

12. **Ardha Chandrasana** (Half Moon Pose)—Inhaling deeply, raise both your arms above your head and tilt slightly backward.

13. **Namaskar** (salute)—Return to stand facing the sun, both feet touching, palms joined together in prayer pose.

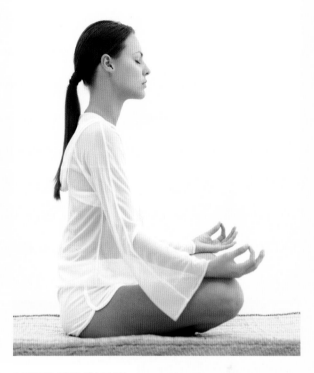

GUIDED MEDITATION

Meditation can give you a sense of calm, peace, and balance that benefits both your emotional well-being and your overall health. And these benefits don't end when your meditation session ends. Meditation can help carry you more calmly through your day, improve certain medical conditions, and even help treat food addiction and help beat cravings.

Guided meditation (or guided imagery or visualization) is a method of meditation where you form mental images of places or situations you find relaxing. You try to use as many senses as possible such as smells, sights, sounds, and textures.

As part of this program, I have created a guided meditation I want you to practice before each meal.

NATURAL BEAUTY

The skin care industry has the public convinced that their products will bring you a glowing complexion, reduce wrinkles, wipe out acne, and turn back the clock on aging. However, it might shock you to learn that the cosmetic industry is not regulated by any formal government organization, and the side effects of these so-called miracle products might be causing more damage than you know! Even many of the products marketed as natural actually contain less than 1% of a natural ingredient such as aloe vera or other essential oils, while still being packed with dangerous chemicals and preservatives.

The United Nations Environmental Program estimates that approximately 70,000 chemicals are in common use across the world, with 1,000 new chemicals being introduced every year. Of all the chemicals used in cosmetics, the National Institute of Occupational Safety and Health has reported that nearly 900 are toxic—although other groups attack that figure as being far too conservative.

And all of these toxins wreak havoc on your body. For example, triclosan is an antimicrobial chemical found in hand washes toothpastes, and household products that has been shown to kill the "friendly bacteria" in our gut that help with digestion and protect the body from more serious infection. There is also cause for concern that the overuse of anti-bacterial products inhibits the normal process of the immune system to ward off germs.

Another example are parabens, which are used as preservatives in cosmetics, food, and house-hold products. These chemicals have been shown to mimic the female hormone, estrogen, and have been linked to an increase risk for breast cancer.

And all of these toxins lurking in your favorite face cream or body wash are going straight onto and into your body. Over time, as the skin tries to cope with these foreign substances, it becomes overburdened and weak. As a result, our bodies become more susceptible to damage by free radicals, dryness, and sensitivities, all of which negatively impact our health and accelerate the aging process. Even some of the active ingredients that are supposed to treat certain problems actually stop the body from correcting these issues naturally. For example, acne cleansers that strip the skin of its natural oils cause the body to produce more oil, thus perpetuating the problem.

In my opinion, the best way to achieve glowing, youthful skin is naturally through proper nutrition, exercise, and minimizing stress. There are some amazing skin boosting foods that you can incorporate into your diet to create a beautiful inside *and* outside!

» **Carrots**—the high beta-carotene content in carrots helps combat signs of aging and can even reverse damage that has already occurred!

» **Eggs**—eggs are high in lecithin, one of the primary building blocks of cell walls, which protects against aging. They are also high in coenzyme Q10, which heightens your level of squalene, which helps keep your skin hydrated and supple. Make sure to eat mostly egg whites to keep support your alkaline diet while keeping cholesterol low.

- » **Green tea**—packed with antioxidants, green tea helps protect your skin against free radicals that cause aging while also providing protection against UV damage. It has also been shown to help your skin cells live longer, d preventing the dull, tired look caused by dead skin cells.

- » **Olive oil and olives**—olives and their oil are rich in oleic, which helps to plump skin, thus reducing the appearance of wrinkles and fine lines.

- » **Pomegranate**—this delicious fruit is packed with age-fighting power, including ellagic acid, which makes your skin heal quicker, antioxidants that protect cells from free radical damage, and even its own form of natural sunscreen that can actually boost your protection from UV light by 25 percent.

- » **Raisins**—raisins are an excellent source of resveratrol, which is a powerful antioxidant that fights aging by slowing down the rate at which your skin cells age.

- » **Turkey (organic)**—on top of the many other health benefits of this holiday bird, turkey boasts high amounts of carnosine, an amino acid that helps prevent wrinkles by protecting the skin's collagen.

Get these superfoods in your insides and watch them go to work on your outside!

SKIN BRUSHING

I know what you're thinking: What the heck is skin brushing? Well, let me tell you.

Skin brushing is a cleansing technique that improves your blood circulation, encourages the elimination of toxins, and supports your lymphatic system. It appears in a wide variety of historical contexts. Athletes in ancient Greece used skin scrapers to improve their circulation and remove sweat from their bodies after contests, while for centuries the Japanese used skin brushing to prepare themselves for traditional hot baths.

Skin brushing can improve your health in a number of ways. For a start, your skin is actually the largest organ in your body. It is often called the "third kidney" because it plays such a vital role in removing toxins from the body, expelling up to a pound of waste a day through its semi-permeable membrane! It is also the place we most often see imbalances that exist in the body coming to the surface. Skin brushing removes the top layer of dead skin cells and encourages new skin cells to grow while unclogging your pores, allowing toxins to leave your body more efficiently.

Stimulating your lymphatic system is perhaps the most important part of skin brushing. The lymphatic system is a crucial part of your immune system, acting as a filter that prevents pathogens from entering your bloodstream. By improving your blood circulation, skin brushing enables your liver to remove toxins more easily.

Lastly (and ladies, I know you'll love this one), skin brushing can be an effective way to treat cellulite! The improvements in blood and lymph circulation, combined with the elimination of toxins under the skin, have been found to help remove at least some of those pesky dimples.

The great thing about skin brushing is that it's a simple, easy-to-understand way to enhance the detoxification process. You can easily fit it into your daily routine before showering or bathing.

So how do you skin brush?

There is a very specific way to skin brush. Try using a natural bristle brush (not one made from nylon or synthetic materials) with a long handle to get to all those hard-to-reach areas. By following this method you will to get the most from your treatment:

» It is best to skin brush before you shower or bathe, using a dry brush. Make sure that your skin is dry to avoid damaging it. I love to skin brush first thing in the morning, but if you don't have time, before bed is ok too.

» Always start in an upward pattern, starting on the soles of your feet, using small circular motions.

» Move to your legs, using long strokes. Always brush toward your chest, following the flow of lymphatic fluid which drains at specific points under your collar bones. Focus on areas with more cellulite a little longer.

» Go counterclockwise on your stomach and abdomen.

» When you move to your arms, start at the fingertips and brush toward your body, using small, circular strokes in your armpits.

» Brush your shoulders and upper chest, always down toward your heart. Use delicate motions in these areas.

» When you are finished, shower or bathe and dry yourself thoroughly.

» I love to finish the process by moisturizing with coconut oil. It smells great (like a trip to the beach!) and is a good antifungal agent to supplement the skin brushing treatment.

For best results, perform this routine daily.

HYDROTHERAPY

If you've ever been to a spa that features a series of pools varying in temperature, you may already be familiar with hot/cold hydrotherapy and its benefits. For those of you who are not, here's the skinny: hot water has relaxing properties, helping to reduce stress, while cold water helps relieve inflammation and stimulates the removal of toxins from elimination organs like the skin and lymph.

Hot/cold hydrotherapy works by subjecting the body to cold external temperatures, directing the flow of circulation inward toward the internal organs. When the temperature changes to hot, the flow of circulation is reversed toward the skin. Alternating hot and cold makes the circulation move in and out like an accordion. This, in effect, moves toxins out of the body and nutrients to various parts of the body. Furthermore, this therapy is also thought to aid weight loss by helping brown fat tissue burn more fat in response to cold temperatures.

And the best part is you can enjoy the benefits of hot/cold hydrotherapy right in your own shower! Here's how:

1. Get completely wet with a temperature of water that is comfortable.

2. Slowly increase the temperature of the water until you can barely stand it. Quickly expose all the parts of the body to this hotter water, including the top of your head and your face.

3. Once this is finished, begin lowering the temperature to the coldest you can stand. Again, make sure all parts of your body get this cold water exposure.

4. Next, increase the temperature again, but try and make it a little hotter than you had it the

first time. Get each part of your body good and hot before reversing the temperature to the coldest possible setting.

5. Repeat the process seven times—seven times hot, seven times cold.

Make sure you always begin with hot and end with cold. If this is too much for you, try simply ending your usual shower with cold water. You will still reap some of the benefits of this therapy.

In a similar vein, it is also effective to splash your face with cold water in the morning and at night to increase circulation, giving your skin a healthy glow! Want an even bigger healthy skin boost? Try switching your nighttime moisturizer for coconut butter or liquid vitamin E. Coconut butter has youth enhancing, glow encouraging properties for the skin, is highly moisturizing, and promotes skin elasticity. Vitamin E provides the skin with necessary moisture as well as antioxidants for intense healing and reduction in the signs of aging. Try mixing it with olive oil for a smoother application and added moisture.

EXFOLIATION

Many of us know the benefits of exfoliation in whisking away complexion-dulling dead skin cells. But it does more than that: exfoliating increases cell turnover to reveal newer, healthier skin cells. Plus, it decreases blackheads, minimizes hyperpigmentation and fine lines, and imparts an all-over healthy glow. It also helps with hydration because as cells transition from below the skin's surface to the topmost layer, they bring with them essential lipids and moisture. And what better time than spring to bust out the exfoliants for the body and feet too?

However, it is important to not take the word "scrub" too literally—especially on the face—because over-exfoliating will result in red, irritated, flaking skin. Instead, gently massage exfoliants into the skin, using light pressure with a washcloth or a loofah. And you can save some big bucks (while keeping your exfoliating routine "clean") by skipping the fancy drugstore products and mixing up an easy homemade skin-softening salt or sugar body scrub from common kitchen ingredients.

As we discussed earlier, department and drugstore beauty products are teeming with toxins and chemicals that cannot only damage your skin, but can cause real health concerns. The best way to avoid exposing yourself to these harmful chemicals is to create your own products at home. And the best part is you'll literally save hundreds of dollars!

Here are some of my favorite at-home hair and skin tonics that will keep your skin glowing and your body toxin-free:

REMEDIES FOR DRY SKIN

Moisture-Charged Face Cleanser

2 oz. vitamin E gel (you can buy them in caps and squeeze out the inside)

1 tsp. jojoba oil

1 tsp. glycerin

½ tsp. grapefruit seed extract

8 drops rosewood essential oil

4 drops rosemary essential oil

Mix all ingredients together in a jar or container and shake well. Apply with a cotton ball or pad and rinse well with warm water.

Sweet Orange and Sesame Nourisher

2 oz. sesame oil

10 drops lemon essential oil

5 drops sweet orange essential oil

5 drops patchouli essential oil

Mix all ingredients together in a jar or container and shake well. Place a few drops of the mixture in your palm along with a few drops of water. Blend and pat gently over your face.

Revitalizing Citrus Cleanser

2 oz. witch hazel

1 tsp. vinegar

1 tsp. glycerin

½ tsp. grapefruit seed extract

6 drops lemon grass essential oil

2 drops tea tree essential oil

Mix all ingredients together in a jar or container and shake well. Apply with a cotton ball or pad and rinse well with warm water.

Cooling Mint Nourisher

2 oz. sesame oil

10 drops peppermint oil

5 drops clary-sage oil

5 drops sandalwood oil

Mix all ingredients together in a jar or container and shake well. Place a few drops of the mixture in your palm along with a few drops of water. Blend and pat gently over your face.

Cleansing Almond Scrub

1 tsp. crushed almonds

½ tsp. powdered milk

½ Tbsp. ground chia seeds

5 drops orange blossom essential oil

Mix ingredients together then add enough water to form a paste-like consistency. Gently scrub over face with circular motions and rinse with cool water.

Flower Power Nourisher

2 oz. sweet almond oil

10 drops sandalwood oil

5 drops rose oil

5 drops geranium oil

Mix all ingredients together in a jar or container and shake well. Place a few drops of the mixture in your palm along with a few drops of water. Blend and pat gently over your face.

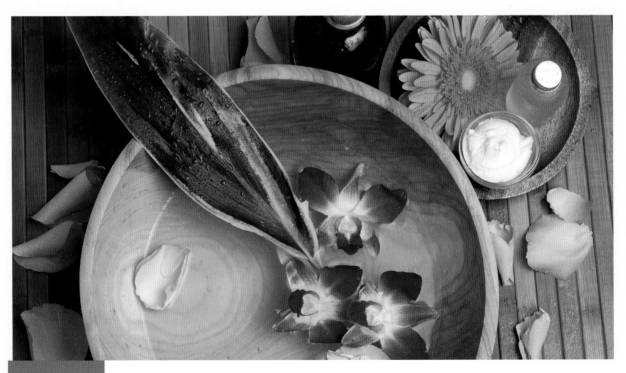

Oatmeal Honey Face Mask

This simple yet effective mask is suitable for all skin types, is super simple to prepare, and will cleanse and rejuvenate your skin in just 10 minutes!

1 Tbsp. oatmeal, finely ground

1 Tbsp. organic plain yogurt with live and active cultures

a few drops of honey (preferably organic)

First, add the yogurt to the oatmeal in a small bowl and mix together. Next, warm a few drops of honey. To do this, warm a spoon under hot water for a minute, then add a few drops of honey to the spoon.

Once warm, stir the honey into the yogurt and oatmeal mixture. Apply the mask evenly over your face and leave it on for 10 minutes, then rinse off with several splashes of warm water. Follow up by patting your skin with a warm washcloth. Finish with your favorite nourisher recipe from above.

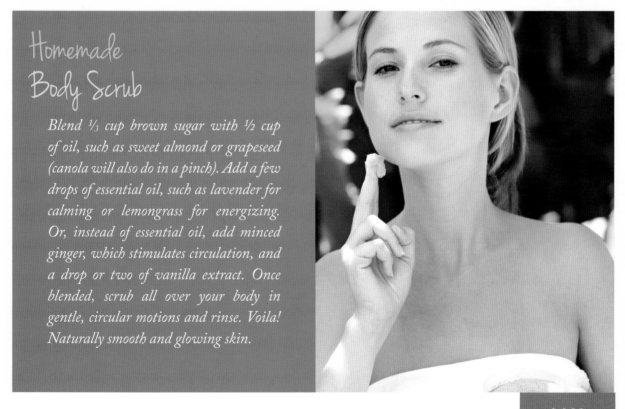

Homemade Body Scrub

Blend ⅓ cup brown sugar with ½ cup of oil, such as sweet almond or grapeseed (canola will also do in a pinch). Add a few drops of essential oil, such as lavender for calming or lemongrass for energizing. Or, instead of essential oil, add minced ginger, which stimulates circulation, and a drop or two of vanilla extract. Once blended, scrub all over your body in gentle, circular motions and rinse. Voila! Naturally smooth and glowing skin.

Deep Conditioning Avocado Hair Mask

Between flat irons, curling wands, blow dryers, and coloring, most of us put our hair through a lot on a daily basis. Dry, brittle, and dull hair is something we all want to avoid, but fancy salon treatments can be pricey (and filled with unknown chemicals). This all-natural hair mask is easily made at home with ingredients you most likely already have in your kitchen.

4 tsp. sunflower oil

1 Tbsp. ground hemp seeds or hemp seed oil

½ ripe avocado

1 tsp. lemon juice

1 egg yolk

Mash the avocado in a bowl. In a separate bowl, whisk together the sunflower oil, lemon juice, and egg yolk. Pour over the avocado and mix well. Spread the mixture over dry hair, and then wrap head in a hot, wet towel. Leave for 30 minutes, and then rinse. You'll be amazed by how smooth and shiny your hair feels!

COLON HYDROTHERAPY

As the last organ to process your food (and its nutrients) before it leaves the body, the colon plays a crucial role in digestion. It is responsible for storing waste for the final eliminatory stage of digestion, the absorption of vitamins (such as vitamin K), maintaining proper water balance, and providing a location for good bacteria (flora) to grow. And perhaps most importantly, it is charged with the task of moving toxic waste and digested food out of your system. When external toxins (those found in our air, our food, our water, and so on) are not properly expelled by the colon, they become internal toxins that are absorbed into our bloodstream and invite the proliferation of harmful bacteria that wreak havoc on our immune system and contribute to a number of health issues including chronic fatigue, inflammation, chronic pain, and even weight gain.

Hydrocolon therapy is a procedure whereby a slow flow of water is released into the rectum in an attempt to clean out any toxic waste. The process does not use any drugs or chemicals, only warm, filtered water is used. With the aid of a trained technician, a small tube is inserted into your rectum while you lie on a table. The water is flushed into your colon, inducing contractions and encouraging the matter inside the colon to be expelled from the body. The technician may massage the abdomen, allowing more matter to dislodge from the colon. The fecal matter gets washed away into a tube and into a sanitary storage area. A typical colon hydrotherapy session lasts about 45–60 minutes, with the amount of sessions recommended varying on an individual basis.

It is important to successfully cleanse the bowel in order to successfully cleanse the body. And the good news is that you can start in your own home. An at-home enema is a great way to start the colon cleansing process cheaply and from the comfort of your own bathroom. Simply follow these easy directions for a cleansing at-home enema:

1. Start with a clean, reusable enema kit.

2. Fill the enema bag with 1 liter of filtered room temperate water. Attach the hose, clamp, and nozzle to the enema bag according to the manufacturer's instructions.

3. Lay a clean towel on the floor to lie on. You may also want a pillow for added comfort.

4. Lubricate the anal insertion nozzle with a generous amount of natural oil (coconut, olive, or almond are best) to ease insertion.

5. Hang the enema bag from your shower curtain bar or cabinet handle, or lay it on the ground 2–3 feet away from where you are lying.

6. Next, slide the clamp down along the tube until it is low enough to be reached from your enema position. Then open the clamp to allow all of the air to escape the tubing.

7. Lubricate your anus with the same type of oil you used to lubricate the enema nozzle. This will allow the nozzle to be inserted with the greatest amount of comfort.

8. Lie down on your towel and assume a comfortable position that affords you easy access to your anus. On your hands and knees with your buttocks in the air is a popular position, while others prefer to lay on one side with one leg stretched straight.

9. With your dominant hand, insert the lubricated nozzle three to four inches into your anus. As you press the nozzle inside, take a few deep, calming breaths to encourage your sphincter to

relax. The nozzle should slide right in, but if you experience resistance, gently twist the nozzle back and forth while easing it inside your anus.

10. Turn on the flow of the enema by opening the clamp slowly. Keep your hand near the clamp in case you need to stop the flow. During your first few enemas, you are likely to experience some degree of cramping as your bowels expand. When this happens, simply stop the flow and allow your bowels a few moments to relax. Similarly, if you feel the need to evacuate your bowels (another common occurrence), simply stop the flow and allow your bowels to relax for a few moments, and then start the flow again.

11. Slowly remove the nozzle from your anus when the enema bag is empty or you feel you can take no more fluid. Ideally, try and hold the liquid for 10–15 minutes (especially if you are attempting to relieve constipation).

12. Move to the toilet and release the fluid.

13. Last, clean your enema kit by mixing a ratio of one part vinegar per liter of water solution. Rinse all parts of the enema bag thoroughly with the solution and allow it to air dry.

DRY SAUNA

Much like a more traditional steam sauna, a dry sauna is an enclosed area where raised temperatures (around 200°F) cause increased levels of sweating. Dry saunas are only used for a few minutes at a time and are often followed by cold showers or baths.

Dry saunas can have many positive health benefits. First, they are very detoxifying, because the profuse sweating allows for the removal of toxins from the body, including cancer causing heavy metals like lead, nickel, and cadmium. It is also great for cardiovascular health, increasing the heart rate and helping to drop diastolic blood pressure, making for a healthier heart. In addition, dry saunas help raise body temperature to create an environment that destroys bacteria while increasing leukocyte levels and boosting the immune system.

They can also help fight signs of aging and promote healthier skin. When circulation is increased, minerals and nutrients are carried to the skin, which helps to grow new skin cells and encourages collagen and elastin production.

Dry saunas can also be extremely beneficial for mental health as well. The warmth of the sauna allows you to breathe deeply, having a calming effect that helps relieve stress. Many also notice a feeling of rejuvenation and renewal following a sauna session. You can increase these effects by adding aromatherapy oils such as calming lavender to the steam to further enhance the relaxation.

It is best to start with short sessions in the sauna of 15 minutes or less 3 times a week until you get acclimated.

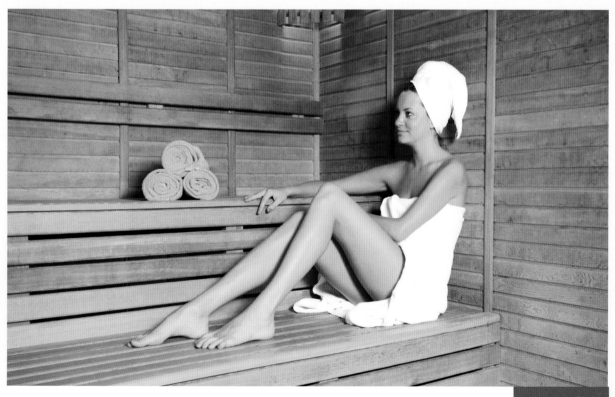

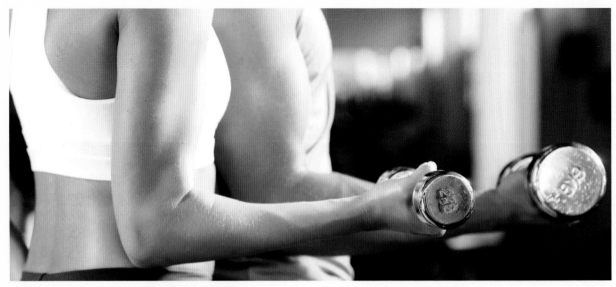

AN ACTIVE CLEANSE

If you want to build an extraordinary life, you have to start by building an extraordinary body. If you want an extraordinary body, you need to make the time each day to build a strong foundation and put your passion and energy into your body. Exercise produces feel good hormones, boosts your metabolism, increases lean muscle, and makes you feel and look great!

When it comes to exercise, most people don't follow through with things because they believe them to be too difficult. They want immediate comfort, and they want the results today! Most people are also full of excuses as to why they can't work out: "I'm too tired,""it's too hard," or "it's too time-consuming." What has happened here is that they have made the "too" TOO big in their own mind. It is their perception that has to change.

To overcome this mind set, you must understand the power of *now* and the power of doing one thing. If you have 20 minutes, or even 10, there is no reason why you can't use that time to get moving! Trust me, getting moving physically will not only build momentum toward a healthier you, but will also build momentum in all areas of your life.

It is true that during a cleanse it is important to give your body the rest it needs while it detoxifies, but a little light activity will not only increase your energy levels, but will actually encourage the cleansing process while creating positive fitness habits.

Below are some excellent options for getting active that are light, fun, and best of all, effective!

Walking—*it's the most simple and natural exercise we do, yet times we forget how beneficial this simple physical act can be. Most of us no longer even think of it as exercise! But trust me—it is, particularly when detoxing. A simple 20–30 minute walk provides a whole host of positive effects, such as loosening up stiff and sore joints and moving important nutrients and oxygen throughout the body by increasing circulation. On top of that, walking helps burn fat, creates glowing skin, enhances mood by getting those endorphins pumping, and increases energy levels. Wanting to kick your walk up a notch? Try power walking by increasing your speed and getting those arms pumping!*

Bicycling—*remember how freeing and fun riding a bike was when you were a child? The wind in your face as you pedaled forward on a warm, sunny day. Well, guess what? It's still that amazing as an adult! In fact, riding a bike is an excellent low-impact exercise for fitness neophytes and veterans alike, and it's particularly perfect during a detox program. A 30-minute bike ride at an easy pace will have a similar effect to walking or jogging while getting your blood pumping,*

oxygenating your body, and getting those nutrients flowing!

Yoga—*this ancient practice that focuses on empowering both the mind and the body has increased in popularity over the past decade—and for good reason. Yoga is linked to an abundance of health benefits. The poses used in a traditional class work to improve posture, increase balance, and sculpt long, strong muscles. But beyond the physical, yoga has also been shown to improve sleep, decrease anxiety, and improve self-confidence due to its inward focus. And the best part is there are different practices that fit any fitness level. If you are already an active person, try a more dynamic Ashtanga class. If you prefer a slower paced class more focused on stretching and relaxation, then Hatha is more for you. Plus, many studios will let you try a class for free before signing up, so what have you got to lose?*

Pilates—*developed in the early 20th century by Joseph Pilates, this low impact body conditioning routine helps build flexibility, muscle strength, and endurance in the legs, abdominals, arms, hips, and back. It puts emphasis on spinal and pelvic alignment, breathing, and developing a strong core or center, and improving coordination and balance. The practice can be adjusted based on level of expertise, making it a great option for both beginners and advanced practitioners. One major reason why people are such big* fans of Pilates is because the practice helps you become more aware of your body, both in and out of the studio, by teaching you how to breathe—useful when you're out on your daily run—and how to stand correctly—useful for making your belly look that much flatter. Ready to grab a mat yet?

Strength/Weight Training—*Strength training is exercising with the goal of increasing your physical strength. There are two kinds of strength: relative strength, which is gaining strength while incorporating cardio so as not to increase body weight; and absolute strength, which is about becoming stronger regardless of body weight. While it's true that aerobic exercise may burn more calories per workout, every additional pound of muscle gained means your body burns around 50 extra calories every day of the week. In fact, research has shown that regular resistance training can increase your Basal Metabolic Rate by up to 15%. And weight training is just as suitable for women as it is for men. It is also suitable (and I recommend it) for people of any age. In fact, it is an excellent way of combating several symptoms of aging. For example, resistance exercise can reduce bone deterioration and build bone mass, preventing osteoporosis, while also inhibiting the effects of sarcopenia, the age-related loss of muscle mass, strength, and function. Furthermore, you can purchase hand weights rather inexpensively and perform routines that work with your own body weight (such as push-ups, squats, lunges,*

and tricep dips), meaning you can have an effective workout at home if you cannot afford or don't have time to go to a gym.

Zumba—*Zumba is a dance fitness method based on salsa and other Latin dance moves, performed to Latin and world music beats, and choreographed to allow people of any fitness or dance experience level to enjoy a fantastic (and fun!) workout that burns a ton of calories and works your entire body. Zumba has been shown to help lower your cholesterol, improve cardiovascular health, and even lower your blood pressure. It also helps improve mood and mental well-being by not only releasing powerful endorphins, but also through the fun and upbeat nature of the music and the social aspect of the class format itself. No matter what your age or fitness level, Zumba lets you dance your way to a cleaner, healthier you!*

Fitness Classes—*When many of us think of fitness classes, we think of neon, spandex, and 80s style workouts lead by big-haired instructors. But group fitness classes are more popular than ever in today's fitness landscape, and with good reason! First, fitness classes are a wonderful place to meet people who have similar lifestyle goals and needs as you, to make friends, to have adult conversations and to discover solutions to problems by talking with other participants. Secondly, participating in a group challenges you to work out beyond your perceived limitations and with the guidance* *and encouragement of the instructor and the other classmates. Also, having an instructor explain the benefits of each exercise increases your reasons to complete the workout and keeps you returning to class.*

And you'll never be bored with the variety of exercise choices offered in group settings. From kickboxing and step aerobics to boot camps and spin, there are so many ways to challenge and improve your body. If your goals are cardiovascular improvement and weight loss, pick aerobic-based classes like Zumba, spinning, or kickboxing. Choose weight training or boot camp classes if you also want to improve your muscular endurance and strength. If flexibility is your goal or you are simply looking for something lower impact, a pilates or yoga class is a great option.

THE DETOX BREATH

Oxygen is one of the most important nutrients in the human body. It is possible for the body to go months without food and days without water, but it can only go a few precious minutes without oxygen before suffocating. We do it so naturally that we don't give it much thought, but breath really is the source of life, and learning how to breathe more deeply and fully is a vital way to keep the body's cleansing and detoxifying systems working at full capacity. The Detox Breath is an effective breathing exercise that acts to strengthen the lungs, massage and tone the abdominal muscles, and refresh the nervous system.

1. Start in a comfortable position. You can stand, sit, or lie down, as long as you feel relaxed and are breathing regularly and normally.

2. Inhale slowly, smoothly, and deeply into the lungs, but do not strain your breathing.

3. Next, exhale all the air out quickly, much like a sneeze. You should notice a contraction in your abdominals as you exhale.

4. Inhale once again as in step 2, smoothly and deeply. This will feel automatic after the quick exhale.

5. Repeat this technique for a few minutes or however long you desire, allowing yourself to relax and focus on your breath. At first, you may find you can only engage in this technique for a minute or so, but as you practice it will become easier.

Special Note: *If you have high blood pressure, any heart condition, epilepsy, hernia, or any ear, nose, or eye problems, I do not recommend you participate in this exercise. If you are pregnant or menstruating, swap the quick exhale for a long, smooth exhale through pouted lips to reduce the intensity of the exercise.*

YOUR FITNESS SCHEDULE

Over the course of the program I would like you to slowly introduce physical activity into your daily routine, increasing the length of the workouts as we progress. Don't worry—I'm not asking you to run a marathon or bike across the country. Just 30 minutes of light physical activity a day can have tremendous benefits to both your mental and physical health. So here's what *I am* asking of you:

WEEK 1

Perform at least 30 minutes of physical activity 3 to 5 times this week. You can do this activity any time of day.

WEEK 2

Increase the length of your sessions to 45-60 minutes. Again, do them at any time of day you choose.

WEEK 3

Introduce one or two 30-minute "fasted" cardio sessions performed first thing in the morning. To make sure you do not burn hard earned muscle, have 1 cup of coconut water mixed with ½ a scoop of iso—whey protein powder—before your session.

WHAT IS FASTED CARDIO?

Fasted (or morning) cardio is a low-moderate intensity cardio session performed before breakfast. By performing cardio before you eat in the morning, you can burn more body fat for energy due to depleted glycogen stores from the 6–8 hours you were asleep (and therefore not eating) and increase your metabolic rate for the day.

Fasted cardio is essential for fast fat-loss because it promotes the use of fat versus carbohydrates for fuel. Let me explain further: when you are asleep, your body burns fat as a fuel. We call them free fatty acids (FFA) because, simply put, they are fatty acids "freed" from your muscle and fat cells. When you wake up in the morning, many FFAs are still delocalized and thus available to be used as fuel (oxidized). If you were to eat breakfast, your body would instead burn any carbohydrates you ingested instead of the FFAs, thus reducing the fat burning potential of your workout.

It is important to note that fasted cardio sessions should be shorter in length, ideally no longer than 45 minutes.

MEAL PLANS

When you're in control and aware in your kitchen, you not only feel better mentally and physically, but you have complete say over what goes into your food. That means less garbage (and excuses) and more wholesome and clean food in your belly.

This program's meal plans were designed with a few things in mind: First, convenience. I have ensured that you get the most of your time by offering cleansing, yet simple meal options that won't take you hours to prepare. Each weekly meal plan also comes with a grocery list of everything you'll need that week, saving you tons of time.

Second is flexibility. As mentioned earlier, I recommend sticking to the program as closely as possible, and that includes eating the foods I have outlined. However, there is always some wiggle room when it comes to allergies or taste preferences, and so I have offered some helpful substitution examples for when the need arises.

Last is your budget! I don't expect you to go broke over the next 21 days, so I have designed the meal plans to fit any budget. I want you to cleanse and de-stress, not have panic attacks over your grocery bill!

You will experience the best results if you follow the plans as I have outlined, and I know you want to emerge from this program cleansed, rejuvenated, and feeling like the best version of you!

So, let's take a closer look at what you can expect over the next 21 days . . .

ADELE'S
Top Ten Detox Rules

1. No dairy produce (except organic, plain yogurt or goat produce)

2. No red meat (except grass-fed beef)

3. No sugar

4. No coffee or caffeinated beverages

5. No jams or spreads (except organic honey)

6. No alcohol

7. No artificial sweeteners

8. Drink 1 to 2 liters (8 cups) of water per day

9. Eat protein with every meal or snack

10. Choose organic (whenever possible)

MORNING CLEANSING DRINK

Each morning, start the day with a cleansing juice or smoothie upon waking. Why? Most studies show that drinking juice in the morning (on an empty stomach and alone) is the best time of day to reap all its benefits because the nutrients will be absorbed more easily when it doesn't have other food to interfere with your body's cleansing. Furthermore, the vitamin-packed fruits and vegetables will not only provide you with the energy needed to start the day, but they will help balance your blood sugars and keep them balanced all day long.

MEAL OPTIONS

Each week I will lay out seven options for each meal and snack you can enjoy throughout the day. You can choose every option once over the course of the week, or repeat some options based on personal preference or allergies. The choice is yours! But each meal or snack option promises to be both detoxifying and delicious!

Because everyone has a different schedule, I have not set out specific times to enjoy each meal or snack. You can eat according to your own personal schedule. However, I advise you to try and eat every 2 to 3 hours, never going longer than 4 hours without food.

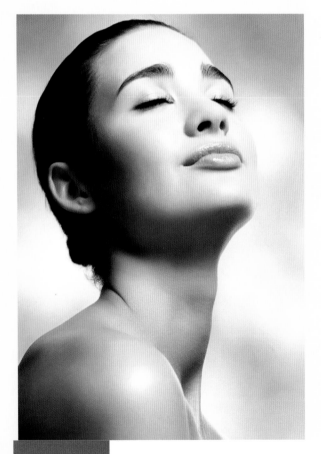

CAVALIERE

The purpose of a detox diet is to allow your liver to rid the body of toxins that have accumulated over time. Some foods can interfere with your body's ability to do this, which is why it is necessary to cut certain foods and drinks from your diet for the duration of the program (and preferably after as well).

I understand that this can be tough for people, so here is a list of foods you should ideally avoid with substitution suggestions that will make eliminating these items easier:

SUGAR—I know you've heard this before, but sugar really is poison for our bodies. But perhaps what you didn't know is that sugar is also sneaky, creeping into our foods under a variety of names, including glucose, fructose (as in fruit sugar), lactose (as in milk), sucrose (as in table sugar), maltose or malts (as in rice malt), jam (contains concentrated juice, which is high in fruit sugar), maple syrup, corn syrup, palm sugar (traditionally used in macrobiotic cooking), and the very deceiving organic brown sugar, which is not all that different from white sugar. Even alcohol is a sugar. All of these sugars are problematic in many different ways. But here comes the good news: We do not have to give up the sweetness of sugar in order to be healthy; we just need to replace it with better alternatives. Here are some natural replacements to help quell those sweet cravings:

» **Stevia**—This plant-based sweetener is not only calorie-free, but in its powdered form, it's 300 times sweeter than sugar, meaning you only need a little for sweetening. It is widely available at many grocery and organic food stores under a few different brand names, including Truvia and PurVia.

» Xylitol—This naturally occurring sweetener, found in the fibers of many fruits and vegetables, is just as sweet as table sugar (sucrose), but has about 40% fewer calories and 75% fewer carbohydrates. That in and of itself can make a big impact on your waistline! Also, xylitol is slowly absorbed and metabolized, resulting in very negligible changes in insulin, therefore avoiding the rise in blood sugar caused by regular sugar, an effect that puts tremendous strain on your system, causing negative health effects. And because it doesn't break down in extreme temperatures like other sweeteners, it's a great substitute for sugar in baking.

» Honey—Honey is natural, sweet, and has a lower GI than sugar, meaning it does not cause the spike in insulin that sugar causes. The types with the lowest GI are floral honeys such as manuka, orange blossom, or buckwheat. It also has antimicrobial properties. However, despite honey being a superior choice to sugar, it is still high in calories and should be used sparingly—no more than one Tbsp. per day.

» Coconut Sugar—Coconuts have become trendy in recent years due to the recent boom in the sale of coconut water that has accompanied a growth in demand for coconut sugar. Coconut sugar is created when sap from the coconut palm is heated to evaporate its water content and reduced to usable granules. It is nutritious and, like floral honeys, has a low score on the glycemic index. It is similar to brown sugar in taste but is slightly richer. You can substitute coconut sugar for traditional sugar pretty much wherever you use the latter.

DAIRY – From a young age we are told that milk is necessary to grow strong bones and prevent osteoporosis. But the truth is that dairy actually causes more health problems than it solves, including acne, anemia, anxiety, arthritis, headaches, heartburn, indigestion, irritable bowel syndrome, joint pain, poor immune function, allergies, ear infections, colic, obesity, heart disease, diabetes, autism, Crohn's disease, as well as breast, prostate, and ovarian cancer. Organic plain yogurt is my one exception to the dairy rule, providing good bacteria that aid greatly in digestion. Instead of your usual 2% or skim, try:

» Unsweetened Almond Milk—Almond milk is one of the most nutritious milk substitutes available. It doesn't contain saturated fats or cholesterol, but it does contain omega-3 fatty acids, so it's very good for your heart. It is also an excellent source of both protein and fiber, is very low in calories (only about 40 calories per one cup serving), and is low in carbs at only two grams per serving. You also get a healthy dose of vitamin E, manganese, selenium, magnesium, potassium, zinc, iron, fiber, phosphorous, and calcium.

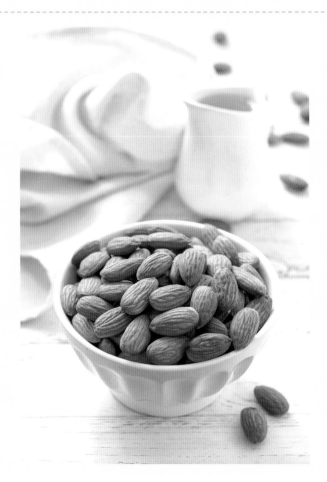

However, when it comes to almond milk, the only healthy option is to make your own. Why? Despite its recent growth in popularity, store-bought almond milk is not the nutritional powerhouse marketers would have you believe. On top of being filled with toxic synthetic vitamins and minerals, your typical carton of store-bought "almond milk" also contains additives, preservatives, and added sugars. Even if you purchase the unsweetened and organic variety, it will still contain harmful chemicals that wreak havoc on your body. Simply put, there is no healthy choice for almond milk that exists on supermarket shelves today. But don't worry—making your own almond milk at home is easy! Here's how:

Organic Almond Milk Recipe

Yield: approx. 5 cups

Ingredients:

2 cups whole raw organic almonds

6 cups water

1 tsp. pure vanilla extract (optional for added flavor)

Other equipment:

juicer (a blender will work too, but a juicer is best)

cheesecloth or fine mesh strainer

Preparation:

1. Begin by soaking the almonds overnight. This will soften them and break down the phytates (antioxidant compounds found in whole grains, legumes, nuts, and seeds that can bind to certain dietary minerals and slow their absorption). Once finished soaking, drain the water from the almonds and discard.

2. Next, run the almonds through your juicer, or if using a blender, blend on low speed with 3 of the 6 cups of water, pulsing so as not to overheat your blender.

3. Lastly, strain the mixture using a cheesecloth or fine mesh strainer into an airtight jar or container, and voila—fresh, chemical-free, homemade almond milk!

Storing: Raw, homemade almond milk will keep for 3–4 days in the fridge. You can freeze any extra almond milk you won't use immediately.

» Organic Hemp Milk—Another great alternative to cow's milk is hemp milk. A vegan product, hemp milk is a blend of hemp seeds and water with a creamy texture and a subtle nutty taste. It's a great alternative for people with lactose intolerances since an allergic reaction to hemp milk is uncommon. It is also easy to digest, has an essential fatty acid balance that is ideal for the human body, is a great source of protein, and contains a plethora of vitamins and minerals. In fact, just one 8-ounce glass contains:

» 900mg omega-3 fatty acid	» Vitamin A
» 2800mg omega-6 fatty acid	» Vitamin E
» All 10 essential amino acids	» Vitamin B12
» 4 grams digestible protein	» Folic acid
» 46% RDA of calcium	» Vitamin D
» 0% Cholesterol	» Magnesium
» Potassium	» Iron
» Phosphorous	» Zinc
» Riboflavin	» And more . . .

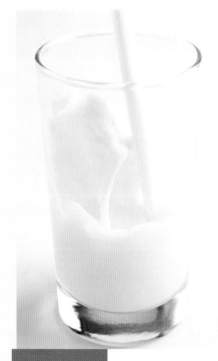

However, like almond milk, it is best to make your own at home to avoid any added chemicals and preservatives that might be lurking in the store-bought variety. Here's how to make your own hemp milk at home:

Homemade Organic Hemp Milk Recipe

Yields: approx. 6-7 cups

Ingredients:

1 cup organic hemp seeds (shelled)
5–6 cups water
natural sweetener such as coconut sugar, stevia, or raw organic honey

Other Equipment:

blender
cheesecloth or fine mesh strainer
glass mason jar

Preparation:

1. Start by combining the water and the shelled hemp seeds in a blender. If you want a more skim milk-like consistency, use more water. If you want a thicker consistency, use less.

2. Next, blend on high for 2–3 minutes, or until you've reached your desired consistency.

3. After blending, you can sweeten the milk by adding the natural sweetener of your choice and blending again. You can drink it thick or strain it through a cheesecloth to remove the large seed particles. *(Bonus tip: the seed pulp can be used as an excellent body scrub, facial mask, or compost!)*

Storing: the hemp milk will stay fresh for 3 days in the refrigerator in a sealed glass jar. Shake well before each use.

» Greek Yogurt—As I mentioned before, plain organic yogurt—especially Greek yogurt—is one of the only exceptions to my no (or at least limited) dairy rule. With a whopping 18 grams of protein per serving, Greek yogurt is a smooth and creamy way to boost the protein content of your diet. It also offers a good dose of bone-building calcium, is low in calories and sugar, and contains half the sodium content of regular yogurt. It also supports weight loss by helping to speed up your metabolism and promoting fat loss.

Furthermore, because Greek yogurt is minimally processed and has not been heat-treated, it contains essential healthy bacteria, including acidophilus and lactobacillus, which improve intestinal health, reduce diarrhea, and even help to prevent vaginal yeast infections.

» Kefir—The other exception to my no/limited dairy rule is kefir. Kefir is a creamy, yogurt-style fermented milk that is chock-full of natural probiotics, making it a healthy digestive system's best friend. It is fermented by kefir grains that contain the bacteria and yeast mixture clumped together with casein (milk protein) and complex sugars. The bacteria and yeast mixture can actually colonize the intestinal tract, a feat that even yogurt cannot match. The yeast in kefir is able to deal effectively with pathogenic yeasts in the body, cleansing and fortifying the intestinal tract and making it more efficient at resisting pathogens.

Kefir is also loaded with vitamins, minerals, and easily digested protein. And it can be consumed by the lactose intolerant! It even works to promote weight loss by reducing food cravings.

And if all that wasn't enough, because kefir is such a balanced and nourishing food, it has even been used to help patients suffering from AIDS, chronic fatigue syndrome, herpes, cancer, sleep disorders, depression, and ADHD.

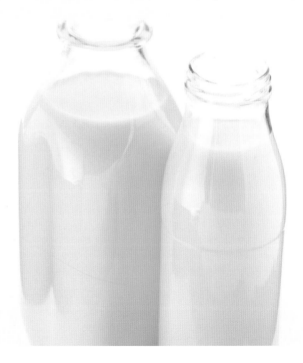

PACKAGED. BOXED. OR CANNED FOOD—Have you ever looked at the label of your favorite canned soup and thought, "What the heck are all these ingredients?" Prepackaged foods are often filled with a plethora of chemicals and artificial ingredients just waiting to wreak havoc on your body, not to mention they are often filled with diet killers like saturated and trans fats, high amounts of sodium, and sugar. It is always better to subscribe to the "clean" method of eating. Clean eating means avoiding processed foods of any kind and instead choosing whole foods in their most natural form, such as fresh fruits and vegetables, whole grains, and local, steroid-free meat and poultry.

If you find it impossible to avoid prepackaged foods, following these easy guidelines will help you improve the quality of your choices:

» Choose options that are simply packaged versions of whole foods, like individual portions of baby carrots, veggie sticks, unsalted natural nuts and seeds, unsweetened oatmeal, natural health food bars, and plain yogurt or cottage cheese.

» Choose options with the shortest ingredient list (aim for three ingredients or less).

» Look for options that have a reduced sodium content.

» Avoid any option where the first, second, or even third ingredient listed is "sugar" (or any of its names).

» Choose organic or low sodium canned vegetables and soups.

TRANS FATS—Trans fats are one of the worst things you can put in your body. Sure, they enhance the taste of your favorite cookies, chips, and frozen pizzas, but once they enter your body, they move into your arteries and turn to sludge. Still sound delicious? The danger is that these trans fats raise LDL "bad" cholesterol and lower HDL "good" cholesterol, greatly increasing your risk of heart disease. To say I highly recommend you cut these from your diet is an understatement. It is one of the best things you can do for your health, and there is no substitution for that!

WHEAT—A wheat-free, or gluten-free, diet has become increasingly popular in recent years. Studies now show that even those who don't suffer from Celiac Disease (a disease where gluten causes an immune reaction that damages the small intestine, causing both great gastrointestinal distress and nutritional deficiencies) can greatly benefit from a wheat-free diet. This is because many of us have a sensitivity to gluten that can lead to similar celiac symptoms such as stomach cramps, diarrhea, and bloating. When it comes to weight loss, one of the quickest ways to drop extra pounds is to cut bread from your diet. This does not mean cutting carbs completely; there are lots of grain options you can still enjoy, such as:

» Quinoa (often called the "super grain" due to its complete protein chain)

» Brown Rice

» Steel Cut Oats

» Amaranth

» Buckwheat

CAFFEINE Caffeine is the most universally used drug, helping you stay alert, improving focus, and even making breathing easier by relaxing airways. Found in many of our favorite drinks, most North Americans consume caffeine daily. But like all drugs, it is addictive and can have negative side effects such as insomnia, anxiety, and adrenal imbalances. If you're someone who adores your morning cup of coffee, or regularly consumes caffeinated beverages throughout the day, you may experience withdrawal symptoms when eliminating caffeine. Symptoms include headaches, tiredness, and irritability. Though this might be a difficult part of your detox program, here are some tips on how to prevent it, or at least lessen the effects:

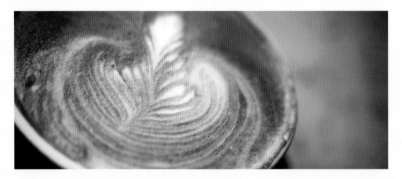

» Gradually decrease your caffeine intake in the two weeks prior to starting the diet.

» Try substituting some of your coffee intake with decaffeinated coffee. For instance, try having a cup of coffee that is 75% regular coffee and 25% decaffeinated coffee. Gradually up the percentage of decaf until you're ready to eliminate it entirely.

» Switch to lower-caffeine green tea, white tea, matcha, or oolong tea.

» If it's the bitter taste of coffee you miss, try a caffeine-free herbal coffee substitute such as Roastaroma tea.

Don't worry. The symptoms of caffeine withdrawal tend to only last a few days, depending on how much caffeine you consume. Just remind yourself that this is your body ridding itself of a harmful toxin, something you can feel good about!

BEDTIME "IMMUNE BOOSTING WEIGHT LOSS" MEAL OPTION

Throughout the meal plans, I have also included a special "before bed" snack option. These are options high in protein, healthy fat, and vitamin C that are designed to aid weight loss and give your immune system a proper boost.

WHY PROTEIN BEFORE BED?

Many of us have heard the dangers of eating before bed in terms of weight gain. And it's true that eating the wrong snack can derail your efforts. That's why it's necessary to choose the right snack. As you sleep, your body steadily gets closer to a catabolic state, which is the process of your body utilizing vital protein and amino acids, the building blocks of protein, as energy. Unfortunately, this process can cause your body to use fat-burning muscle as a source of fuel. By eating a high-protein snack right before bedtime, you can help to slow down this process and make sure your body is properly fed throughout the seven or more hours you sleep, meaning your muscles will stick around to burn fat another day!

WHY HEALTHY FATS AND VITAMIN C BEFORE BED?

Healthy fats (like omega-3s) are essential for normal growth and development. Dietary fat also provides energy, protects our organs, maintains cell membranes, and helps the body absorb and process nutrients. Even better, it helps the body burn fat! Furthermore, studies show that when your diet is deficient in omega-3s, production of melatonin (the sleep hormone) is thrown off, resulting in less sleep, which as we know is imperative to a weight loss plan. Add in the immune-boosting power of vitamin C and you've got a pre-bedtime recipe for a restful and reparative sleep.

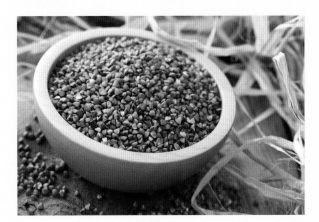

THE 21-DAY DETOX PLAN—
LET THE CLEANSING BEGIN!

You are about to embark on a life-changing journey toward perfect health, a more empowered way of living, and ultimately a more empowered you. Are you pumped? Wave-your-arms-above-your-head-while-doing-an-embarrassing-dance excited? You should be! If you truly commit to this program and the goals you want to accomplish over the next 21 days, you will emerge with a renewed sense of positivity, joy, and well-being. Just do the very best you can and know that I have total faith in you!

This program is not designed to force you into a cookie-cutter plan that doesn't allow you to experience it in the way that works best for you. But I don't want to leave you entirely without guidance either, which is why each day will include a sort of "detox to-do" list to guide you through the program and help you achieve the best results possible. Your Daily Detox To-Do will include the following:

» A Morning Cleansing Drink—Most studies show that drinking juice in the morning (on an empty stomach and alone) is the best time of day to reap all its benefits because the nutrients will be absorbed more easily when it doesn't have other food to interfere with your body's cleansing. Furthermore, the vitamin-packed fruits and vegetables will not only provide you with the energy needed to start the day, but they will help balance your blood sugars and keep them balanced all day long. I will make a daily suggestion, but feel free to refer to the recipe section for your deliciously juicy options.

» Daily Prep—Staying organized and prepared is crucial to staying on track, so each day I advise you to prepare your meals for the day as much in advance as possible. This includes having all tools and equipment (Tupperware, water bottle, and so on) ready to go. Refer to page 3 for a refresher on how to prep and stay organized. This also involves choosing which recipes you are going to enjoy that day. Refer to your meal plan on pages 160–161 for all your tasty options.

» Daily Affirmation—The purpose of this program is not to simply detox your body, but also restore a sense of mental well-being and positive self-image. Your daily affirmation is a message you repeat to yourself starting first thing in the morning and carry through the day to help you stay motivated and improve your overall attitude and outlook on life. Refer to page 110 for a deeper look at positive affirmations.

» Tip or Trick—Life gets busy, money gets tight, schedules get off course—such is life! But each day I will let you in on my little secrets for staying on track no matter what life throws your way.

» Lifestyle Upgrade—These tasks may include incorporating a new food into your diet, drinking more water, performing a fitness challenge, or trying a new mental exercise such as meditation—any task that will improve your life either physically, mentally, or spiritually. Each task is designed to help you achieve that overall perfect health you are looking to create over the next 21 days.

» A Detox 101—It is important that you leave this journey with the necessary knowledge to carry the changes you have made in this program into the rest your life moving forward. By understanding the reasons behind the various elements of each detox day, you will be taking full responsibility for your own health, which is a not only vital for your 21-day journey, but for the rest of your life.

At this point I'd also like to refer you back to the "Getting Started" section of this book on page 8) as a refresher on what you need in order to begin. You may want to refer back to this section often to help you stay organized and on track. If you have made the decision to work out at home instead of at a gym or fitness class, you may also want to invest in the following items:

» Jump rope

» Handheld weights

» Yoga/Pilates mat

Okay, let's recap: Healthy foods? Check! Running shoes? Check! Positive attitude? Check! Ok then—let's get started!

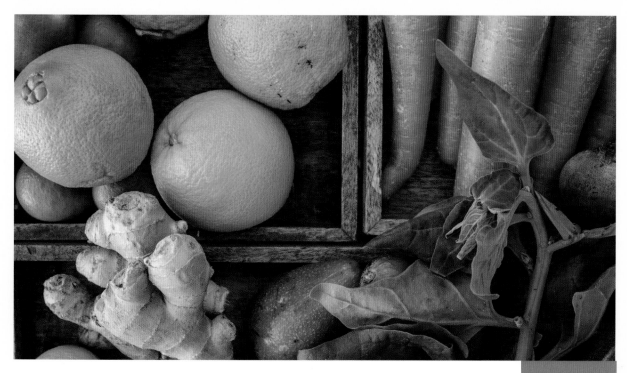

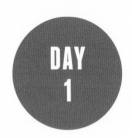

DAY 1

Welcome to Day 1! This really is the first day of the rest of your healthier and more vital life. By now, you should have everything you need from your checklist and have performed all the necessary tasks in order to get started. Your pantry should be purged; your kitchen should be stocked and organized; all tools and equipment, such as water bottles, Tupperware, and a blender/juicer, should be acquired; and your fitness clothes, fitness bag, and running shoes should ready by the door. Staying organized is incredibly important. Taking 20 minutes the night before or early in the morning will ensure an easy, fun, and positive day. Commit to doing this for each day throughout this program and success will be that much closer!

DAILY AFFIRMATION

"Every cell in my body vibrates with energy and perfect health. I am in control of my mind and body and I nourish my soul with my positive, powerful thoughts."

DAILY PREP

Get chopping, get packed, and get organized!

TIP OR TRICK

Prepare emergency snacks! This way if something comes up or you miss a meal, you always have a healthy option on hand to stave off the hunger monster! Fruits, veggie sticks, pre-washed/packed salads from the grocery store, natural nuts and seeds, and protein shakes are some excellent options.

LIFESTYLE UPGRADE

Start drinking lemon water throughout the day. For the next 21 days (and hopefully every day after), ensure you are drinking at least 2 liters of water per day. As a detoxifying bonus, include fresh lemon or lemon juice in your water bottles and drink throughout the day.

MORNING CLEANSE DRINK	BREAKFAST	MID-MORNING SNACK	LUNCH	MID-AFTERNOON SNACK	DINNER	EVENING SNACK (OPTIONAL)
Refreshing Cucumber Basil Juice (p. 129)	Rise and Shine Shake (p. 113)	We Got the "Beet" Juice (p. 129)	Cucumber Salad with Mint (p. 141)	Choose 1 Snack Option	Choose 1 Dinner or Entree Option	Sleepy Time Smoothie (p. 157)

DAILY 101:

LEMON + WATER = BEST OF FRIENDS

Water is life. It makes up more than two-thirds of our body weight and is paramount to the proper functioning of our bodies. It regulates body temperature, aids in proper digestion, lubricates our joints, transports valuable nutrients to our body, and, of course, carries harmful toxins out of it. This is why increasing your water intake is a crucial component of any detox program.

As you cleanse and detoxify your body, you will be releasing the toxins, bacteria, and viruses that

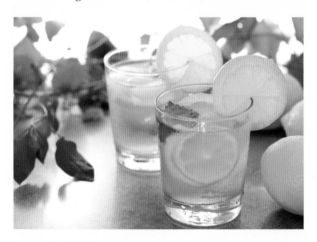

were built up in your body over the years. As they are released, you may experience symptoms of past illnesses that have left their mark in your body through the toxic deposits they left behind. You may get a runny nose, feel tired and experience body aches. You may even develop a fever. But these will

be temporary and are simply your body's response to the release and flushing out of these toxins.

By drinking water, you are encouraging and speeding up the removal of these toxins. And as an extra detoxifying step, I want you to drink your water with lemon.

Lemons contain a plethora of vitamins and minerals that help your body detoxify and aid weight loss efforts. First, they are high in vitamin C, which helps regulate the body's insulin production and supports the metabolization of carbohydrates, which greatly helps control cravings (something you will appreciate as we move forward in the program). Vitamin B12, found in lemons, plays a role in converting fat to carbohydrates and vice versa, while vitamin B3 helps with the metabolization of unsaturated fatty acids, carbohydrates, and cholesterol, helping to support digestion and prevent gastrointestinal disorders. A lemon's magnesium content helps with the normalization of potassium, phosphorus, calcium, adrenaline, and insulin levels, all of which support body functions related to maintaining a healthy weight. And lastly, lemon juice is a diuretic, helping to flush undesirable bacteria and toxins out of the body while also eliminating water weight. Ready to pour a glass yet?

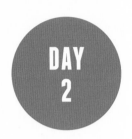

DAY 2

You've made it through your first day, so let's keep the momentum going by touching on a very important component of success in this journey: staying accountable. Simply put, being accountable means being honest with yourself and acknowledging where you've succeeded, and where there is room for improvement. The best way to do this is to keep a mood and food journal in which you track your meals, your fitness efforts, and your emotions to better understand the progress you are making and where you might make changes to better your results. It also gives you the opportunity to reflect on the achievements you made that day and celebrate your hard work. Woo hoo!

DAILY AFFIRMATION

"I love and accept myself. I understand and accept that my imperfections makes me perfect. Therefore, I am perfect exactly as I am and will remain perfect as I learn and grow."

DAILY PREP

Get chopping, get packed, and get organized!

TIP OR TRICK

Want to find fresh, organic produce at a fraction of the cost of store prices? Find your local farmers market! See page 14 for more information on the many reasons to shop local.

LIFESTYLE UPGRADE

Get journaling! Studies show keeping a fitness, food, and mood journal doubles your chance of success and is essential to helping you stay motivated and accountable. It is crucial that you write in your journal each and every day of this program. This is your story of transformation and it's worth telling!

MORNING CLEANSE DRINK	BREAKFAST	MID-MORNING SNACK	LUNCH	MID-AFTERNOON SNACK	DINNER	EVENING SNACK (OPTIONAL)
A Forest of Fiber Juice (p. 130)	Choose 1 Breakfast Option	Weight Loss Tonic: Green Juice with Grapefruit (p. 133)	Choose 1 Salad Option	The Craving Crusher (p. 119)	Cellulite Crusher Greens Salad (p. 144)	Choose 1 Late-Night Immunity Booster Option

Simply by joining this program, you have made a commitment to change your life. But it's important to truly understand what it is you want to achieve and why you want to achieve it.

I want you to start by closing your eyes. What does your success look like? Are you comfortably zipped into a favorite pair of jeans? Are you energetically chasing your children around the park? Are you walking down the street wearing a confident smile? Are you finally free of a specific health issue?

By understanding the results you want, you are one step closer to successfully achieving them. You have the power to make this vision a reality.

Next, you must organize how you're going to achieve it, and this starts with getting organized. Organize your thoughts, your schedule, your pantry, and, of course, your goals. As the age-old adage goes, "People don't plan to fail. Instead, they fail to plan." Today, I want you to establish a clear plan for success.

CREATE YOUR PLAN OF ACTION

An effective action plan lays out the changes, steps, and actions you will need to take over these 21 days to achieve your goal. A good action plan is clear and often includes the answers to the following questions:

» What actions or changes will occur?

» Who will carry out these changes?

» By when they will take place, and for how long?

» What resources (i.e. money, equipment, support) are needed to carry out these changes?

An action plan is fluid and may change over the course of your 21 days, so don't lock it away in a drawer and forget about it. Keeping it visible will not only let you amend it when necessary, but will also help you to remember what you're working toward.

CREATE YOUR GOALS

In this exercise, you will write down both your short-term and long-term goals, focusing on your ideal future and how you will motivate yourself to get there. This should happen on 3 levels:

» First, you create your "big picture" goals: What do you want to do with your life over the next 10 years? What are the large-scale goals that you want to achieve?

» Next, break these down into smaller and smaller targets that you must hit to reach your lifetime goals.

» Finally, once you have your goals set, you start working toward achieving them.

CREATE A FOOD, MOOD, AND EXERCISE JOURNAL

Research shows that keeping a written account of your weight loss efforts doubles your chances of success, mainly because it holds you accountable. You're far less likely to eat that cookie when it's going to stare at you from a page for the rest of the day. And on the other side of the coin, seeing all your progress is extremely encouraging, motivating you to keep moving forward. This week, I want you to start your own journal, tracking your meals, moods, and physical activity.

Over the next 21 days, I want you to revisit your action plan and your goals, and to then write in your journal every day. Keeping these things in mind will help you remember what you are working toward, making success that much more attainable. See page 185 for a template to help you get started.

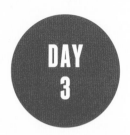

DAY 3

Day 3 already! How are you feeling so far? I hope by now you're feeling a little more energized, a little more focused, and even more excited about the changes you will see over the course of this journey. I am your cheerleader, your coach, and your teammate—and I know you can do this!

DAILY AFFIRMATION

"I can accomplish anything I set my mind to, and I set my mind to becoming physically and mentally fit. I am physically fit and I am mentally fit."

DAILY PREP

Get chopping, get packed, and get organized!

TIP OR TRICK

Looking for a simple (and tasty) way to rev your metabolism and boost your immune system? Add freshly-ground, natural spices to your food whenever you can. Start by adding some ginger, turmeric, or garlic to any of your cleansing juices, or sprinkle some cinnamon into your morning oatmeal or smoothie.

LIFESTYLE UPGRADE

Get up and get moving! Starting today, try and include 30 minutes of physical activity in your day, every day, preferably first thing in the morning. No need to make it too intense or complicated to start. Try a morning walk outside or on the treadmill, or, one of my personal favorites, take an invigorating morning yoga class.

MORNING CLEANSE DRINK	BREAKFAST	MID MORNING SNACK	LUNCH	MID AFTERNOON SNACK	DINNER	EVENING SNACK (OPTIONAL)
"Get Glowing" Skin Renewing Juice (p. 131)	Calcium Smoothie (p. 118)	We Got the "Beet" Juice (p. 129)	Choose 1 Lunch Option	Choose 1 Snack Option	Choose 1 Entree Option	Choose 1 Late-Night Immunity Booster Option

Adding spices and dried herbs to your food not only adds a punch of flavor, but it can also provide valuable health and weight loss benefits. Filled with antioxidants, minerals, vitamins, and unique medicinal properties, let's take a look at three spices in particular that will take any meal (and weight loss plan) to the next level!

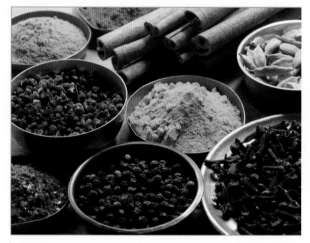

TURMERIC

If you're a fan of curry, you already love the unique and aromatic flavor of turmeric, the yellow-orange spice that makes the foundation of many curry dishes. Though you may be familiar with its flavor, you may not know all of the amazing health benefits that accompany it. Curcumin, one of turmeric's most thoroughly studied active ingredients, reduces the formation of fat tissue by suppressing the blood vessels needed to form it, and therefore may contribute to lower body fat. It may also be useful for the treatment and prevention of obesity-related chronic diseases such as insulin resistance, hyperglycemia, hyperlipidemia, and other inflammatory symptoms associated with obesity and metabolic disorders.

GINGER

Ginger is another warming spice that has anti-inflammatory properties and is known to help soothe and relax your intestinal tract. Research also suggests that ginger may have thermogenic properties that help boost your metabolism, and also has an appetite-suppressing effect when consumed. Adding a pinch of this amazing spice to a smoothie or in a detox soup will kick up the flavor and your weight loss efforts!

GARLIC

The healing properties of garlic have been harnessed for thousands of years (a Sanskrit record from India mentions its medicinal properties 5,000 years ago), but it can also play a major role in encouraging weight loss. Through its more than 100 biologically helpful compounds, garlic boosts your metabolism, is a powerful detoxifier, eliminates fat from the cells, is an effective diuretic, and regulates sharp ups and downs in your blood sugar levels (causing carb and sweet cravings as well as fat storing). And the added bonus is that it's delicious. So go ahead and season soups and other meals generously with this incredible spice.

This week I want you to incorporate these powerful spices into any meal you can.

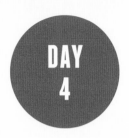

DAY 4

One reason why people don't always realize their full potential is because they are trapped in the past and are afraid of letting go. Make an effort today to release those negative emotions and perceptions that might be holding you back from making the positive change you seek. The future is yours to shape; make it the amazing life journey you deserve.

DAILY AFFIRMATION

"I know that the world is shifting to bring forth everything I desire. I now see opportunities, I now have ideas, and I now have the means to accomplish my goals."

DAILY PREP

Get chopping, get packed, and get organized!

TIP OR TRICK

Nature provides tons of ways to create beautiful skin without harmful chemicals. Try using natural ingredients like shea butter for a more even skin tone, tea tree oil for inflamed acne, and witch hazel to calm redness. Just add a few drops to your nighttime moisturizer!

LIFESTYLE UPGRADE

Removing sugar from your diet may seem scary, but it could be the one thing that is holding you back from achieving the goal you have always wanted to accomplish. What other habits, attitudes, or beliefs might be holding you back? Today, I want you to create of list of all the things that may be limiting you from reaching your full potential. Next, create a plan for overcoming these obstacles. You are the master of your own destiny, and you are in control!

MORNING CLEANSE DRINK	BREAKFAST	MID-MORNING SNACK	LUNCH	MID-AFTERNOON SNACK	DINNER	EVENING SNACK (OPTIONAL)
Workout Wonder Juice (p. 128)	Choose 1 Breakfast Option	Choose 1 Juice Option	Choose 1 Salad Option	Citrus Wheatgrass Juice (p. 125)	Choose 1 Entree Option	Choose 1 Late-Night Immunity Booster Option

DETOX 101: SEE YA LATER. SUGAR

Sugar, or as I call it "white poison," is an addiction. Most of us don't realize it, but we are sugar addicts! We use sugar even when we don't know we're doing it. It's in salad dressing, peanut butter, soup, pickles, bread, jam, yogurt, and canned fruits and vegetables, and we crave it after every meal. On average, each of us consumes about 130 pounds of sugar per year.

And this substance is also devoid of any nutritional value. Sugar passes through the wall of the stomach so quickly that it causes blood sugar levels to skyrocket, then plummet just as rapidly. I'm sure you are familiar with the feeling.

Because it is literally everywhere, beating your sugar addiction may seem like a hopeless battle. But just like any addiction, you have to have a structured plan to win the war. Here are my top tips for beating sugar cravings:

1. Stick to foods that are closest to their original form.

2. Eat protein with every meal.

3. Read labels!

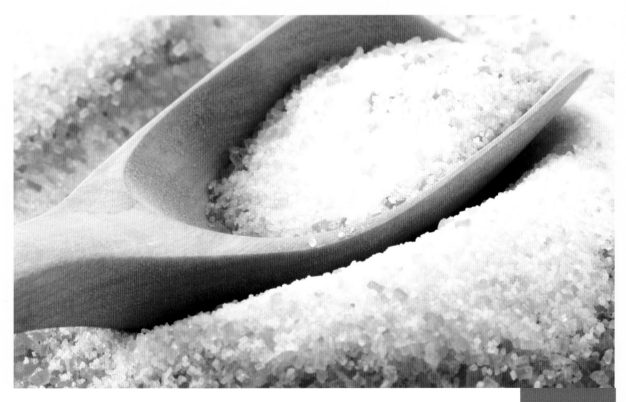

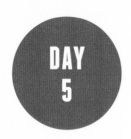

DAY 5

Most of our lives are plagued by one nagging question: How can I make room for my own well-being when there aren't enough hours in the day? We all know that our lives are jammed packed, but are we creating extra work and obligations for ourselves by thinking we're more essential than we actually are? Break free from the endless demands and accept that you can't do it all. Take time for yourself and return to the world with a renewed sense of calm and positivity.

DAILY AFFIRMATION

"My body is amazing and I love my body. In order to show the deep love and respect for my body, I choose to eat healthy foods. Each moment I decide to eat or drink something, I am conscious of the impact it will have on my overall health and I make healthy choices."

DAILY PREP

Get chopping, get packed, and get organized!

TIP OR TRICK

A quick protein shake is an easy and delicious way to sneak more protein into your diet, even when you're on the go. Blend one up in the morning and pour it into a portable container for a protein-packed meal or snack, no matter where your day takes you.

LIFESTYLE UPGRADE

Earlier in this book we talked about how important meditation is to reducing stress, improving your relationship with yourself, and increasing your overall sense of well-being. Guided meditation is an excellent option for newbies. Gabrielle Bernstein's *May Cause Miracles* guided meditation album is one of my personal favorites, but there are many free options available on YouTube. Today, I want you to take at least 15 minutes to settle into the calm and nourish your spirit!

MORNING CLEANSE DRINK	BREAKFAST	MID-MORNING SNACK	LUNCH	MID-AFTERNOON SNACK	DINNER	EVENING SNACK (OPTIONAL)
Tummy-Warming Tonic (p. 128)	Lean Muscle Fruit n' Protein Pancakes (p. 123)	Choose 1 Juice Option	Choose 1 Lunch Option	Choose 1 Juice Option	Choose 1 Dinner Option	Choose 1 Late-Night Immunity Booster Option

DETOX 101: THE POWER OF PROTEIN

Protein is undeniably linked to success in weight loss. In fact, the moment it leaves your fork, protein goes to work slimming your waistline. High-protein foods take more work to digest, metabolize, and use, which means you burn more calories processing them. They also take longer to leave your stomach, so you feel full sooner and for a longer amount of time.

So how do you make sure you're getting enough? Experts advise consuming between 0.5 grams and 1.0 grams of protein per pound of your body weight.

Skew on the high end if you're really active, and on the low end if you're trying to lose weight. If both apply, shoot for an amount somewhere in the middle.

Starting today, I want you to add protein to every meal and snack. Examples of lean protein include chicken, turkey breast, salmon, tilapia, white fish, nuts, seeds, legumes (such as lentils), egg whites, plain yogurt, or pressed cottage cheese.

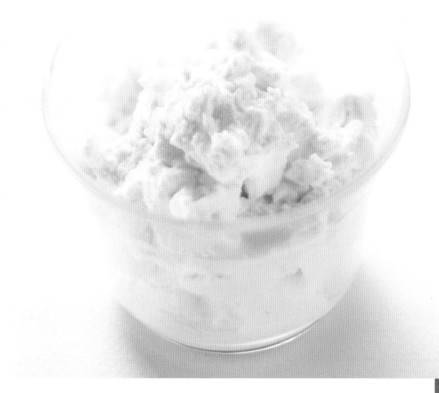

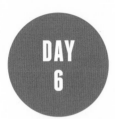

DAY 6

Most of us suffer from a condition I like to call the "need to please" disease, often saying yes to people's requests for our time or energy, even when that yes causes us great stress or discomfort. Although it may feel uncomfortable to say no, it's important to remember that each time you say yes to someone or something else, you say no to you and your priorities. Take a few minutes today to contemplate the following: If you could say no to someone or something, knowing that there would be absolutely no hard feelings or negative consequences, who or what would you say no to? Is there a project you would give up? A relationship you would end? A date you might break? At first, saying no might create some internal guilt. But the tough choices you make today will help you reach a happier place tomorrow.

DAILY AFFIRMATION

"I am in control of my world and my body. I am responsible for myself. I release this unnecessary stress and allow my body and mind to relax into a comfortable state of being. I am calm and relaxed. I have a positive and optimistic mental attitude."

DAILY PREP

Get chopping, get packed, and get organized!

TIP OR TRICK

One of the major mistakes people make is waiting too long between mealtimes. Long stretches without food makes people crave energy-dense carbs (pass the bread basket, NOW!) and can make it difficult for people to make healthy choices and watch portion sizes when they do eat. It may also compromise metabolism. Make an effort to eat every 3–4 hours to keep you metabolism revved and your hunger in check.

LIFESTYLE UPGRADE

If you're not already doing so, start incorporating omega-3s into your diet on a daily basis. The easiest way to do this is to begin taking a fish oil supplement, but adding omega-3-packed foods like salmon or eggs into your diet is also fantastic way to reap the benefits of these amazing, healthy fats!

MORNING CLEANSE DRINK	BREAKFAST	MID-MORNING SNACK	LUNCH	MID-AFTERNOON SNACK	DINNER	EVENING SNACK (OPTIONAL)
Green Apple Wheatgrass Juice (p. 125)	Choose 1 Smoothie Option	We Got the "Beet" Juice (p. 129)	Beet, Avocado, and Kelp Salad (p. 143)	Choose 1 Snack Option	Walnut, Fig, and Lentil Detox Salad (p. 146)	Choose 1 Late-Night Immunity Booster Option

DETOX 101: GET THOSE OMEGA-3S

Over the years, fat has acquired a bad rap, but the truth is not all fats are created equal. Omega-3 fats offer a plethora of health benefits, like lowering cholesterol, improving mental health, and even improving your skin. A healthy diet should include daily servings of these amazing fats, with an emphasis on lean fish like salmon, tuna, or mackerel. You can also find omega-3s in flax seed, olive oil, many nuts, and avocados. Add any of these things to a daily salad and do your body a world of good!

In regards to weight loss, an omega-3 supplement is a great way to ensure you reap all the benefits these fats have to offer. Omega-3 helps with weight loss simply by reducing your insulin levels throughout the day. When insulin levels are high, you can't use fat for fuel. Furthermore, when insulin levels are high, your HGH levels are low. You want HGH to be high and insulin levels to be low, and omega-3 supplements make that happen. Fish oil also directly increases the oxidation of fat within fat cells. Try taking a supplement that has at least 600mg of DHA daily.

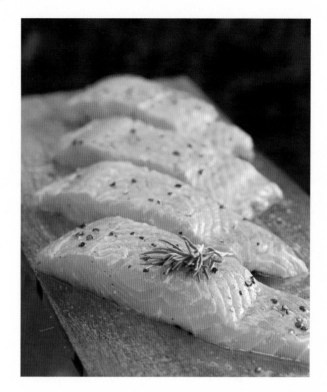

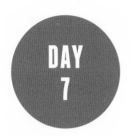

DAY 7

Congratulations! You've completed your first week of this exciting journey! Woo hoo! (Picture an explosion of fireworks, cheers, and standing ovations.) How do you feel? By now, your energy should be on the rise, your moods more balanced, your eyes a little brighter, and your pants (fingers crossed) a little looser! Keep up the amazing work you've done so far and you'll be leaving your unhealthy past sucking your dust in no time!

DAILY AFFIRMATION

"I love myself. I take it easy and enjoy all there is around me. I enjoy nature, I enjoy life, and I enjoy my family. I make the time to spend with each of them regularly and I feel amazing."

DAILY PREP

Get chopping, get packed, and get organized!

TIP OR TRICK

When overhauling your diet to cut out the bad and to embrace the clean and nutritious (as we are doing during these 21 days), cravings for sugar and other old junk food favorites are inevitable, but your giving in doesn't have to be! Food cravings are like any other craving—they only last for a few minutes. When a craving hits, try taking a quick walk, doing some deep breathing, or run through your goals in your mind. Once you have successfully survived the craving, you can bask in the deep satisfaction of beating it, which is far more rewarding than giving in! You can also try my amazing "The Craving Crusher" juice.

LIFESTYLE UPGRADE

Time to take your new body measurements and photos! How far have you come since Day 1? Are you happy with your progress? Are there things you would like to do better next week? Try creating a weekly goal list and outline what you want to accomplish in the week to come. Do this as part of your journey toward success and the healthier, happier life you deserve.

MORNING CLEANSE DRINK	BREAKFAST	MID-MORNING SNACK	LUNCH	MID-AFTERNOON SNACK	DINNER	EVENING SNACK (OPTIONAL)
Red and Tangy Goddess Juice (p. 131)	Protein-Packed Asparagus Omelette (p. 124)	Choose 1 Snack Option	Choose 1 Salad Option	Tummy Warming Tonic (p. 128)	Choose 1 Entree Option	Choose 1 Late-Night Immunity Booster Option

DETOX 101: CONQUERING CRAVINGS

Quitting junk food is like quitting any other addiction, complete with all the cravings. An important goal in this detox process is to reprogram your palate and your system. Instead of demanding immediate gratification from sugar or salt, or a stimulant like caffeine, we want it to settle for a gradual release of whatever it is your body wants from healthier sources, like sugar from carrots or salt from natural seeds.

Another important thing we want to accomplish during this program is differentiating between healthy and unhealthy cravings. Sometimes our body is asking for something because it actually needs it. For example, after a workout, you may crave salt to replace the salt lost during exercise. But instead of reaching for a bag of chips, try some natural corn chips or some crunchy almonds. The trick is to squash these cravings the right way in order to get your body off the rollercoaster of sugar spikes and varying salt levels. We are attempting to achieve balance, and by introducing slow releasing sugar and salt foods, you will eventually rid yourself of pesky junk food cravings for good!

One way to defeat cravings is by tracking them. Tracking your food cravings allows you to better understand them, and, when possible, try to avoid the culprits. Today, I'd like you to start tracking your cravings in your journal, noting the culprits and the frequency. It may also be effective to track the successful ways you dealt with them to use when dealing with future cravings. If it's sugar you're missing, remember to revisit the paragraph on sugar substitutions earlier in this program.

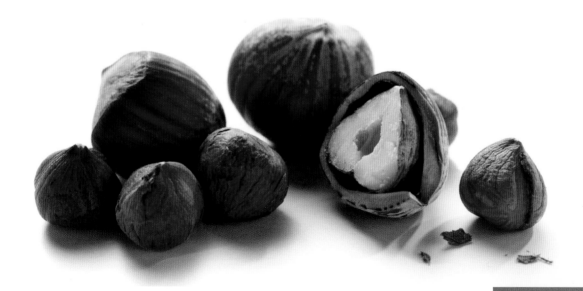

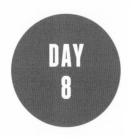

DAY 8

Exercise slumps happen to the best of us. But while getting stuck is inevitable, staying there isn't. One easy way to get unstuck is to respect your body clock. For example, if you run faster at 8:30 AM than at 7:30 AM, the sensible thing to do is move your workout to the later time. Many of us tend to squeeze in activities when we can instead of when we'll achieve the best results. Try listening to your internal body clock and ditch that workout rut.

DAILY AFFIRMATION

"I trust my body and know that it will naturally adjust to an ideal weight for me. Food is nourishment and I make good and healthy eating choices based on my nourishment needs. I move regularly and enjoy every moment of it. I am healthy and slim!"

DAILY PREP

Get chopping, get packed, and get organized!

TIP OR TRICK

By now, performing at least 30 minutes of exercise should be part of your daily routine, but have you incorporated any strength training yet? Everyone, no matter how young or old, should be doing some kind of regular strength training. And doing it at home is easy! Resistance bands and balls, small hand weights, water, and even your own body weight can be used as resistance when designing a strength training program. As a special bonus, ex-NFL star and celebrity trainer Marc Megna has prepared both an at-home and gym-based strength training routine for beginners to help you get started. Visit page 162 to get lifting, and don't forget to record your reps!

MORNING CLEANSE DRINK	BREAKFAST	MID-MORNING SNACK	LUNCH	MID-AFTERNOON SNACK	DINNER	EVENING SNACK (OPTIONAL)
Belly Bloat-Beating Juice (p. 130)	Cardio Apple and Beet Juice (p. 134)	Wheatgrass Shot (3 oz.)	Heart Booster Pomegranate Salad (p. 145)	Water Retention Juice (p. 132)	Choose 1 Dinner or Entree Option	Sleepy Time Smoothie (p. 157)

LIFESTYLE UPGRADE

Get cooking—in class! Taking healthy cooking classes can be extremely helpful in a number of ways. As a hobby, cooking can make your lifestyle cheaper by arming you with the knowledge and know-how to create meals using ingredients that are on sale or left over in your fridge. Cooking at home also gives you full control over what goes into your food, thus limiting the bad fats, chemicals, sugars, and other harmful ingredients found in many take-out or processed meals. You will also learn healthy cooking techniques such as steaming, which can help you prepare food without draining its nutrients. Embrace your inner chef and become the kitchen goddess (or god) you were meant to be!

DETOX 101: BYE BYE BREAD, HELLO FLAT TUMMY!

One of the quickest and most common ways people lose weight today is simply by cutting breads and pastas from their diet. And while it's true that eating too much of anything will cause weight gain, the problem with bread and pasta is that it's very calorie dense, most containing anywhere from 70–80 calories per ounce, meaning it doesn't take long to reach your calorie allotment for the day. Compound that with the fact that most breads and pastas on the market today are made with refined flour, which cuts down on the nutritional value and the fiber content. And as discussed earlier, the less fiber a food has, the more of it you'll eat in order to feel full.

Another problem with breads and pastas is that they tend to be high on the GI scale, meaning that as soon as they hit your bloodstream, they cause a spike in your blood sugar levels. This in turn causes your brain to signal to your pancreas to secrete more insulin. Insulin brings your blood sugar back down, but primarily by converting the excess sugar to stored fat. Also, the greater the rate of increase in your blood sugar, the greater the chance that your body will release an excess amount of insulin and drive your blood sugar back down too low, meaning that in no time you're hungry again!

Your task for today is simple: no breads or pastas. Instead, enjoy a steaming bowl of quinoa or brown rice, or mix up a delicious smoothie or juice. Just remind yourself why you are on this journey and I have no doubt you can successfully complete this small challenge.

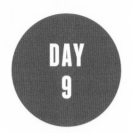

DAY 9

Hopefully by now the clouds of any detox symptoms are clearing and you are starting to feel the warm sunshine of vibrant health on your face. If you are still feeling any emotional, mental, or physical symptoms of detoxing (including irritability, headaches, and mood swings), hang in there! This is completely normal and soon you'll be free of the sludge that has accumulated over the years and feeling like the clean, energized goddess you were born to be!

DAILY AFFIRMATION

"I have every bit as much brightness to offer the world as the next person."

DAILY PREP

Get chopping, get packed, and get organized!

TIP OR TRICK

Now that we're a little ways into your detox journey, let's test your PH levels. It's best to either test 1 hour before eating or 2 hours after. It is also a good idea to test 2–3 times in a day in order to get an average, as first thing in the morning the body has retained fluids and will engage in different processes to remove acid wastes from the body throughout the day (depending on activity and diet). See page 10 for a refresher on how to get testing.

LIFESTYLE UPGRADE

Go under the needle—the acupuncture needle that is! This ancient Chinese practice that focuses on restoring the proper flow of energy and flow through your body has amazing results in treating a variety of ailments, from back pain and sciatica to headaches, nausea, and asthma. It's also been proven effective in treating emotional and psychological disorders. Even if you don't suffer from a specific issue, treatment can strengthen general constitution and can correct a feeling of being "unwell," though there is no physical disorder, imbalance, or illness in the traditional Western medicine sense. So go ahead and balance your Qi!

MORNING CLEANSE DRINK	BREAKFAST	MID-MORNING SNACK	LUNCH	MID-AFTERNOON SNACK	DINNER	EVENING SNACK (OPTIONAL)
We Got the "Beet" Juice (p. 129)	Muscle-Building Spinach Juice (p. 135)	Weight Loss Tonic: Green Juice with Grapefruit (p. 133)	Choose 1 Lunch or Salad Option	Water Retention Juice (p. 132)	Cellulite Crusher Greens Salad (p. 144)	Choose 1 Late-Night Immunity Booster Option

DETOX 101: PROBIOTICS

Our bodies are hosts to trillions of bacteria (the majority living in the colon), most of which are vital in maintaining good health. The friendly bacteria that aid in digestion are called intestinal flora.

The two important groups of flora are the lactobacillus acidophilus, found mainly in the small intestine, and bifidobacterium, found primarily in the colon.

There are many important functions performed by intestinal flora, including:

» Aiding in the digestive process

» Producing B-vitamins

» Producing lactic acid (known as lactic acid bacteria—end product of fermentation as a result of glucose metabolism)

» Producing Vitamin K (aids in blood clotting)

» Producing chemicals that heal the large intestine and counteract the bad bacteria

» Providing natural protection against infection

When these flora are out of balance, it can cause a plethora of issues, including Chronic Fatigue Syndrome, Irritable Bowel Syndrome, obesity, and depression. So how do you make sure they stay balanced?

Probiotics are "good" bacteria that help balance the levels of good versus bad bacteria in our gut. By fighting off disease-causing bacteria, probiotics help support a healthy digestive system and replenish good bacteria in the gut flora, helping combat gastrointestinal infections and bowel diseases.

The best source of probiotics is organic yogurt with live cultures, but you can also find them in a bottled capsule form as well. Starting today, try incorporating at least one serving of organic probiotic yogurt into your diet. If you are lactose intolerant or do not eat dairy, then the capsule form is a possible substitute.

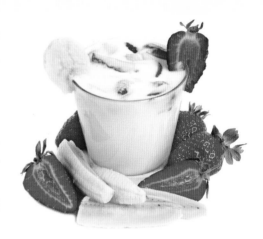

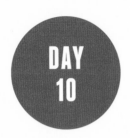

DAY 10

You're at the halfway mark! How are you feeling? Many people begin to experience moments of heightened well-being—even euphoria—due to the mood-boosting foods you've been feasting on the last 9 days. Bask in these moments and feelings, and remember them as your move forward toward a lifetime of love and happiness.

DAILY AFFIRMATION

"I am healthy and happy and I choose to partake in healthy habits only. I choose health."

DAILY PREP

Get chopping, get packed, and get organized!

TIP OR TRICK

Have you been writing in your journal every day? How about reflecting on your progress as you move through this journey? It's important to take the time to celebrate your achievements—victory dance recommended—and to acknowledge where you can improve. Only by truly understanding where you are and where you want to be can you get to your desired destination. Take some time today (and each day moving forward) to consider what you can do to ensure your successful finish!

LIFESTYLE UPGRADE

Take your workout to the next level and schedule a session with a personal trainer. There are many benefits to making this investment, such as improving your form to maximize results and avoid injury, designing a workout to meet your specific goals, learning new skills, expanding your fitness knowledge, and that all-important motivation for sticking with it and pushing past your comfort zone! Just make sure you find the right trainer for you. Ask a friend, talk to your gym's manager, or look online for good reviews. There are even trainers who offer at-home sessions for those who don't have a gym membership. Trust me—making this small investment can make a big difference!

MORNING CLEANSE DRINK	BREAKFAST	MID-MORNING SNACK	LUNCH	MID-AFTERNOON SNACK	DINNER	EVENING SNACK (OPTIONAL)
Water Retention Juice (p. 132)	Weight Loss Tonic: Green Juice with Grapefruit (p. 133)	Bone-Builder Juice (p. 132)	Choose 1 Lunch or Salad Option	½ cup plain yogurt mixed with 1 tsp. ground flax	Choose 1 Salad Option	Choose 1 Late-Night Immunity Booster Option

DETOX 101: POSITIVE AFFIRMATIONS AND VISUALIZATION

We've all heard it: the voice inside our heads that seems to spew a stream of hurtful thoughts, telling us we aren't good enough, smart enough, doing enough. This is called negative "self-talk," and it is the ultimate saboteur to achieving the happy, healthy, and joyful life you deserve. Positive affirmations are the key to silencing the inner critic by replacing negative thoughts with empowering ones. In fact, developing a positive mind set is one of the most powerful life strategies there is. By using positive thinking techniques, visualizations, and positive affirmations, it is possible to achieve whatever you want simply because you believe you can!

Today, I want you to create your own set of positive affirmations. Post them around your home, your work, or wherever you will see them daily. If you're not sure where to start, there are some great examples of good positive affirmations off to the right.

Through the hustle and bustle of this busy world, it's important to carve out some space where you can simply relax, centering yourself and visualizing the change you want to see. Today, I also want you to carve out a space in your home where you can take some time for yourself and sink into the quiet. Buy some scented candles, soft pillows, and some soothing music to help create the ambiance. Spend at least 15 minutes a day in this space, reflecting and being mindful.

I choose to feel good right now.

I choose to trust in the process of life.

I give myself time to recoup and regroup, digest and integrate, by not overcrowding my schedule.

I commit to seeing my beauty and divine essence every time I look in the mirror.

I am in the process of making positive changes.

Step by step I am on the upward path to my goal of (insert your goal here).

I love and accept myself completely, just as I am.

I give myself permission to be healthy, happy, prosperous, and at peace.

I am tapping into the unlimited abundance of the universe.

I now give and receive freely.

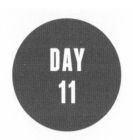

DAY 11

If we want to, we can always find a reason not to do the things we either want to do or know we should do in order to achieve our goals and give ourselves the happiness and health we deserve. There are a plethora of excuses we offer up: "I'm too busy," "I will do it tomorrow when I can really commit," "It's too late for me to change," "I don't have the energy right now." The truth is we all have the same number of hours in a day, and we all have the potential to use them to achieve the things we truly want in life. While it's true it might be easier for some, it is possible for all of us. The key is to acknowledge that your dreams are worth the effort—you're worth the effort—and to be willing to be creative with your resources so you can achieve all you desire.

DAILY AFFIRMATION

"I imagine myself as someone who has already overcome my challenges. I picture a successful resolution in my mind and then observe its appearance in my life."

DAILY PREP

Get chopping, get packed, and get organized!

TIP OR TRICK

Just like strengthening a muscle, meditation and positive visualization get easier with practice. Commit to a daily practice and enjoy the peace and mindfulness that comes with a deeper connection to yourself. Try this technique today to really connect with yourself on a higher level:

Settle into your sacred space, mentally conjure forth a soothing setting, and meditate on a chosen positive affirmation while practicing some deep breathing. Be present in your mental scene with as much detail as possible, focusing on all your senses. What does the air smell like? Is it warm? Is there a gentle breeze caressing your skin? What sounds are around you? Repeat your chosen affirmation as you feel the warmth and safety of the positive mental space you've created. Sit for 15 minutes, enjoying the peace and relaxation.

MORNING CLEANSE DRINK	BREAKFAST	MID MORNING SNACK	LUNCH	MID AFTERNOON SNACK	DINNER	EVENING SNACK (OPTIONAL)
Bikini Body Fruit Juice (p. 134)	Sweet Cherry Almond Oatmeal (p. 123)	½ cup plain yogurt mixed with 1 tsp. ground flax	Choose 1 Lunch or Salad Option	Water Retention Juice (p. 132)	Choose 1 Salad Option	Cooling Nighttime Cucumber Juice (p. 159)

LIFESTYLE UPGRADE

Today's upgrade is simple: Make an effort to go to sleep one hour earlier than usual. Not only does getting a quality night's sleep improve your overall mood, it also supports weight loss efforts by improving metabolic function and can help stave off disease by boosting immune function. Ready for a warm glass of milk and your pjs yet?

DETOX 101: CATCH THOSE ZZZZS

More often than not, people fail to make the connection between good sleep habits and weight loss, but quality sleep is a vital component of any successful weight loss endeavor. Sleep and weight loss studies indicate that if you sleep more, you will weigh less. (In a recent study, researchers in Chicago found two hormones, leptin and ghrelin, were identified as having an influence on appetite, fat storage and cravings.) Ghrelin, which is produced in the gastrointestinal tract, stimulates appetite, while leptin, produced in fat cells, sends a signal to the brain when you are full. When you don't get enough quality sleep, leptin levels drop, which means you don't feel as satisfied after you eat. Lack of sleep also causes ghrelin levels to rise, which means your appetite is stimulated and you want more food. These two factors combined can set the stage for overeating and cravings. In fact, the study also found that when

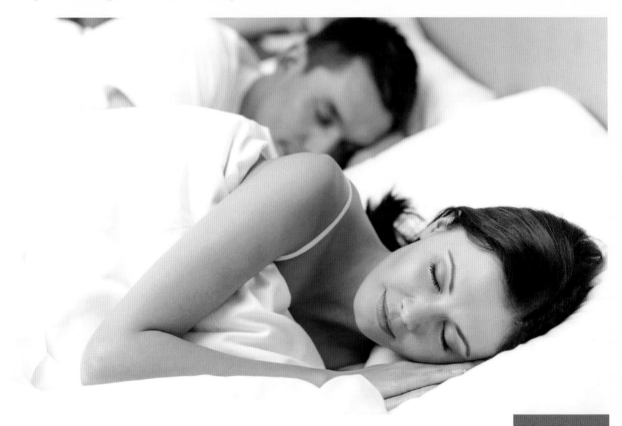

leptin levels dropped due to sleep deprivation, the subject's desire for high carbohydrate and calorie-dense food rose by a whopping 45 percent!

Now, I am by no means suggesting you give up exercise and eating well to sleep the day away so you can achieve your weight loss goals. However, I do recommend making your sleeping patterns a priority to boost your immune system, keep your hormonal system in check, and lose or maintain your desired body weight.

To achieve a proper amount of quality sleep, it is best to start implementing a nighttime pattern. Like most other areas of life, our systems respond best when they get into a routine. Although there will be times and stressers in your life that knock you off your sleep routine, try to implement the following sleep habits into your life to help establish a healing and well-rested sleep pattern:

1. Avoid caffeinated beverages such as coffee, tea, pop/soda, or green tea less than five hours prior to bedtime.

2. Avoid eating high Glycemic Index foods prior to bedtime.

3. If you must eat in the evening, try to select a protein source or a low Glycemic Index carbohydrate.

4. Keep your room as dark as possible.

5. Avoid shift work whenever you can.

6. If you feel anxious about sleeping or suffer from insomnia, try putting lavender on your pillowcases or sheets. Lavender's aroma is relaxing and will help you ease into a peaceful slumber.

7. If you smoke, quit. In addition to being one of the biggest aging elements to your skin and loading your body with free radicals, smoking can also upset sleep patterns.

8. Avoid watching the news or reading the newspaper prior to bed. On an unconscious level, the images can imprint on your brain and psyche and cause a disrupted sleep pattern.

9. Once in bed, record in a journal your day's events and the things for which you are grateful. In a strange way, writing down your thoughts, goals, or most personal dreams has a calming and peaceful effect on the mind.

10. Avoid over-the-counter or prescribed sleep medications. If you need some help falling asleep, try natural sleep aids such as valerian root (available at health food stores), melatonin, or chamomile tea.

11. Eat foods high in tryptophan and calcium (such as turkey, spinach, and kale) to help you get to sleep.

12. Go to sleep and rise at the same time every day. Do not sleep in on weekends; this will only upset the routine you are trying to establish. Ideally, do not go to sleep later than 10 PM.

13. Avoid drinking alcohol before bed.

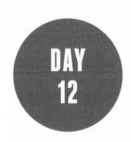

DAY 12

Fridays can be a little scary. With the weekend comes temptation and a break from the weekday routine that helps you stay on track. But your new lifestyle doesn't have to mean deprivation from the traditional weekend fun of friends and festivities. Celebrate your two-day vacation with non-alcoholic cocktails and fresh veggie tapas, then remind yourself that this journey isn't about depriving yourself—quite the opposite. You're giving yourself the greatest gift possible: perfect health and spiritual well-being.

DAILY AFFIRMATION

"I give thanks that I now create vibrant health within my mind and body every day."

DAILY PREP

Get chopping, get packed, and get organized!

TIP OR TRICK

Looking for a natural way to exfoliate? Try a Kiwi! Yes, this delicious tropical fruit not only tastes great, but its seeds make the perfect face scrub. Simply spoon out the green fruit and mash it in a bowl. Once done, rub the mashed fruit gently over your skin and rinse. So simple!

LIFESTYLE UPGRADE

There is an inextricable link between being grateful and being happy. Being grateful reminds us of the positive things in our lives, of what's important, and of those people in our lives who make it a better one. Plus, it costs nothing to be grateful! Take 2–3 minutes each morning to give thanks to whoever or whatever you're grateful for. You don't have to do anything other than close your eyes and silently give thanks. This one act can make a huge difference and give you a warm fuzzy to carry with you all day long.

MORNING CLEANSE DRINK	BREAKFAST	MID MORNING SNACK	LUNCH	MID AFTERNOON SNACK	DINNER	EVENING SNACK (OPTIONAL)
Cardio Apple and Beet Juice (p. 134)	Weight Loss Tonic: Green Juice with Grapefruit (p. 133)	1 brown rice cake topped with 1 tsp. natural nut butter and ground cinnamon	Beet, Avocado, and Kelp Salad (p. 143)	½ green apple 2 mini cucumbers	Choose 1 Dinner Option	1 cup chamomile tea 1 cup celery sticks

Earlier in the program, we touched on cravings and how to effectively overcome them. But sometimes our relationship with food goes beyond simple cravings.

Food addiction is a very real issue for many Americans. Unlike food cravings, it's a behavioral disorder, much like substance abuse or compulsive shopping. The problem is that, unlike luxury goods or narcotics, we need food to survive, making food addiction that much more difficult to treat and ultimately overcome. And with side effects like obesity, psychological distress, and other life threatening health issues, it can have devastating consequences if not treated.

So when does a big appetite and a love of food (good and bad) cross over into the addiction category? Here are some tell-tale signs of compulsive eating:

» You are thinking about the next meal when you are still eating the current one.

» You can't pass by a grocery store or restaurant without stopping to buy your favorite food item.

» The owner or salesperson of a store or eatery knows your usual.

» You buy a dessert or meal accompaniment (such as bread) and eat it as soon as you get home instead of waiting for the meal.

» Sometimes you eat what you bought in the store where you bought it, in the street, or in your car because you're unable to wait.

» You have gradually increased your consumption over time, meaning you eat much more now than you did a year ago, two years ago, and so on.

» You have an increased "tolerance" for food. For example, it now takes eating two donuts to feel satisfied, instead of only one.

» Your behavior continues despite the consequences, such as weight gain or other associated health problems.

If any of this sounds familiar, you may have an addiction to food. So how do you treat it? Addiction takes control of the brain, causing the sufferer to be controlled by the substance, in this case food. Decision-making, motivations, and behavior are all controlled by food. Therefore, the only way to treat the issue is to regain control. It will be hard, but not hopeless! Admitting that help is needed is the first step.

This help will more than likely need to come from a mental health professional, such as a psychologist, psychiatrist, or addictions counselor. And like all addictions, there are certain steps you will have to take to overcome it, including:

Detoxing—*creating a new diet that is bland and simple is the first and most important step of recovery. Eliminating refined foods like simple sugars, flours, many fats, and salt will be necessary for a while in order to overcome the cravings, giving you a chance to regain control.*

Removing Cues—*like any addiction, the preferred substance (in this case certain foods) needs to be made unavailable, or as unavailable as possible. This means the home needs to be cleansed of all foods you have a tendency to overeat. This is because* these foods may cue binges and threaten success in overcoming the addiction. Any other members of the household need to support this step as well.

Re-establishing a healthy pattern of eating—*after years of abuse, a food addict will have established very irregular eating patterns. They may sometimes skip meals just to end up overeating at other times that are unusual to the rest of us. Therefore, a major part of treatment will be developing a regular pattern of eating, most often focusing on 3 main meals and 2 small snacks. Oftentimes, an alarm is used to remind the individual to eat at scheduled times, helping to "reset" their dietary clock to a more normal pattern.*

Getting the right support—*most addicts find it beneficial to connect with others who have the same problem. While family and friends can try to help and offer support, it is good to have a peer group who truly understands what the addict is going through and whom he or she can vent to and discuss challenges with.*

Writing it down—*journaling can be so beneficial for many reasons, but it is extremely beneficial when it comes to recovering from addiction. Stress and other negative emotions can often trigger a relapse. Keeping a journal of eating patterns and moods is a helpful step to gain*

an understanding of how different moods and emotions affect behavior.

Getting active—*developing a regular fitness routine is a particularly effective component of treatment because it not only prevents stress and encourages endorphin production (those chemicals in the brain that make us feel good), but it has also been shown to reduce food cravings, increase eating self-control, and reduce addictive behaviors. (Not to mention the associated weight loss that is most likely necessary after years of overeating.)*

Getting your life back—*Lastly, recovery involves creating a more values-driven, goal-oriented life. Addictive behavior is all about instant gratification and short-term thinking, slowly moving the individual further away from desires in the long-term. Counseling involves creating a plan of action that is consistent with one's values and goals in life, thus driving them toward a more meaningful life that is not dictated by food.*

Because we tend to be addicted to foods that are processed, artificially colored and flavored, and generally bad for our bodies, a diet focused on whole, clean, and detoxifying foods is extremely important. When we rid our bodies of these toxins and slowly remove the culprits from our diet, our body "resets" itself, and we no longer crave those foods that wreak such havoc on our bodies and our lives. Over the course of this program, you are working toward doing just this. It can be hard, but the payoff is worth its weight in healthy, vibrant years!

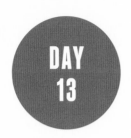

DAY 13

In order for relationships with others to truly flourish, we must first commit to perfecting the ones we have with ourselves, and that requires knowing who we really are. While there is a natural tendency to find an identity in our roles in life (our personality, our work, our body, our culture, our stories of the past, and our dreams for the future), in reality, these are all temporary, external aspects of ourselves. Who we really are is eternal and unbounded. Our true self is pure love and pure spirit. This simply means that truly knowing yourself isn't about searching for anything outside of ourselves. It's about discovering the love that is already within us.

DAILY AFFIRMATION

"Deep at the center of my being is an infinite well of love."

DAILY PREP

Get chopping, get packed, and get organized!

TIP OR TRICK

Sticking to a raw food diet isn't easy. It's best to ease yourself into the lifestyle by starting off slowly. Get yourself started by preparing some snackier foods ahead of time before you dive in completely. Flax crackers, raw granola, or dehydrated fruit can be lifesavers when you need something to hold you over. Making a meal plan, even if you only loosely follow it, can also relieve some of the daily pressure that can accompany a new diet and lifestyle. It saves you time at the market and time spent standing around the kitchen wondering what you're in the mood for.

MORNING CLEANSE DRINK	BREAKFAST	MID MORNING SNACK	LUNCH	MID AFTERNOON SNACK	DINNER	EVENING SNACK (OPTIONAL)
Muscle-Building Spinach Juice (p. 135)	Choose 1 Breakfast Option	Workout Wonder Juice (p. 128)	Choose 1 Salad Option	½ cup plain yogurt mixed with 1 tsp. ground flax	Walnut, Fig, and Lentil Detox Salad (p. 146)	Sleepy Time Smoothie (p. 157)

LIFESTYLE UPGRADE

Have you ever had a stranger pull over to help you change a flat tire? Or let you go ahead in line at the grocery store when you were in a hurry? How good did that random act of kindness make you feel? Science shows that kindness is directly linked to less stress, an increased sense of inner peace, and overall better health. Studies even show that those who perform more random acts of kindness lead a longer and more satisfied life! Plus, they give you the feel-good vibes that come with knowing you helped make someone's day a little bit sunnier. Spread the love and sunshine by making random acts of kindness part of your everyday life!

DETOX 101: GET RAW

As discussed earlier in the program, the benefits of raw food are many.

Dishes prepared with raw foods taste wonderful because the flavors are natural to the foods themselves. They also require fewer additives like salt, spices, oils, and sweeteners. They also have more nutrients and fibers, as they haven't lost any of their vitamin and nutrient content during a cooking process. They are also digested easier, usually taking 24-36 hours as opposed to the 48–100 hours cooked food takes. This saves a lot of energy!

Furthermore, the nutrients found in raw foods strengthen the immune system, thereby preventing illness and disease. A raw diet has been shown to improve the health of those suffering from arthritis, asthma, high blood pressure, cancer, diabetes, digestive disturbances, menstrual problems, allergies, obesity, psoriasis, skin conditions, heart disease, diverticulitis, weakened immunity, depression, and hormonal imbalances.

And if all that wasn't enough, a raw diet causes degenerative diseases to virtually disappear; aging slows, the whites of your eyes become whiter, you have more energy, and you need less sleep.

Today, I'd like you to try and eat only raw foods. If that is too much for you, make at least two meals and any snacks raw. All of the juice and smoothie recipes found in this program are raw, so pick the ones that speak to you and enjoy the fresh and vibrant flavors nature has to offer!

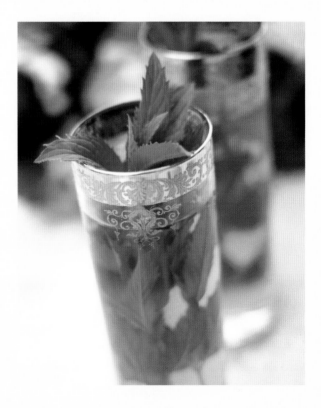

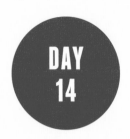

DAY 14

Break out the balloons and streamers, because it's time to celebrate your second successful week of this journey! This is an amazing accomplishment, and if you haven't already given yourself a giant pat on the back (maybe even an enthusiastic fist pump), then please do so right now! You should be proud of your achievements and the positive changes you've made so far. So give yourself a much deserved round of applause—I sure am!

DAILY AFFIRMATION

"I cannot change what I refuse to confront. I confront my challenges with the knowledge that I have the power to change them into possibilities."

DAILY PREP

Get chopping, get packed, and get organized!

TIP OR TRICK

It's progress photo time again! In order to get the best photos possible, pick an uncluttered spot for your photo shoot, either in front of a wall or in front of a door. It also helps to take the photo in portrait mode instead of landscape—you want to see your changing body from head to toe and close enough to see those new muscles! Pssst, don't forget to take fabulous new measurements to accompany those fabulous new photos.

MORNING CLEANSE DRINK	BREAKFAST	MID-MORNING SNACK	LUNCH	MID-AFTERNOON SNACK	DINNER	EVENING SNACK (OPTIONAL)
Weight Loss Tonic: Green Juice with Grapefruit (p. 132)	Choose 1 Breakfast Option	Choose 1 Snack Option	Choose 1 Salad Option	1 brown rice cake topped with 1 tsp. natural nut butter and ground cinnamon	Choose 1 Salad Option	Choose 1 Late-Night Immunity Booster Option

LIFESTYLE UPGRADE

When it comes to health, hormones have a much bigger effect than many people realize. In fact, unbalanced hormones can destroy health even if everything else (diet, supplements, and so on.) is optimized. Conversely, balancing hormones can do a lot to boost health, even if not all the other factors are optimal. And the good news is this can be done naturally with a few simple changes to your diet and lifestyle. Start today by simply cutting out harmful saturated fats found in products such as vegetable oil, peanut oil, soybean oil, margarine, shortening, or other chemically-altered fats. Instead, choose fats like coconut oil, canola oil, and olive oil (don't heat), and eat lots of high omega-3 fish. Read today's Detox 101 to discover more natural ways to get those hormones balanced.

DETOX 101: BALANCING HORMONES

Hormonal imbalances don't just take a toll on you mentally; they can actually sabotage your weight loss efforts. When our hormones are imbalanced, it usually manifests as abdominal fat, which is not only the hardest to get rid of, but also brings the most health risks. The most common hormone imbalances contributing to belly fat are: high estrogen, low testosterone, low DHEA (a hormone of the adrenal glands), high insulin, and high cortisol.

Re-balancing your hormones can be achieved with a few simple actions:

1. De-stress your life. High cortisol levels are directly related to stress, so take a deep breath, increase your exercise, or sink into the couch with a good book. The method doesn't matter as long as you relax!

2. Switch to organic. A lot of today's foods contain harmful chemicals that affect our body's natural hormone balance. Choose organic dairy, meat, and locally grown fruits and vegetables whenever possible.

3. Catch some Zs. Sleep deprivation can lead to increased cravings for sugary and carb-laden foods. Good sleep patterns help weight loss efforts by controlling the hormones that influence appetite and increase metabolism. Try and get 7.5–9 hours of sleep a night to help stay balanced.

4. Bring on the protein! A high-protein diet helps lower insulin levels, the hormone that tells our bodies to either use sugar as fuel or store it as fat. Try and consume 20–25 grams of protein at each meal, and 15–20 grams per snack.

5. Start a supplement. No matter what imbalance you are suffering from, there are numerous health supplements you can take to tackle it. Relora is an herbal supplement that has been shown to aid weight loss efforts by lowering cortisol and raising DHEA.

Today I want you to start rebalancing your hormones by implementing at least two of the above actions into your daily routine. As you begin to feel more balanced and your jeans a little looser, I promise you will soon be enthusiastically implementing them all!

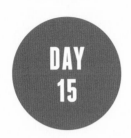

DAY 15

As you prepare for your last week of this 21-day adventure toward perfect health, I want you to take time to reflect on the transformations you've experienced so far—large or small. How has your vision of yourself changed since you began this journey? What shifts have you noticed in your life and in your relationships? How has your mental and physical well-being improved? Recognizing all the positives that have accompanied your dedication to this journey is the best way to stay motivated right to the finish line. Keep up the amazing work!

DAILY AFFIRMATION

"My body is amazing and I love my body. In order to show the deep love and respect I have for my body, I choose to eat healthy foods. Each moment I decide to eat or drink something, I am conscious of the impact it will have on my overall health and I make healthy choices."

DAILY PREP

Get chopping, get packed, and get organized!

TIP OR TRICK

Read the label! Some foods may not taste salty but are actually loaded with sodium. Try to restrict your consumption of foods with more than 600mg of sodium per serving, and limit your total sodium intake to 2300 mg per day. The easiest way to do this is to cut out most prepackaged foods, most of which are teeming with excess sodium. But when you can't, check nutrition labels and choose options that fall within a healthy limit.

MORNING CLEANSE DRINK	BREAKFAST	MID-MORNING SNACK	LUNCH	MID-AFTERNOON SNACK	DINNER	EVENING SNACK (OPTIONAL)
Bone-Builder Juice (p. 132)	Choose 1 Salad Option	1 cup fresh berries, plain	My Good Greens Salad (p. 146)	Choose 1 Smoothie Option	Choose 1 Dinner or Entree Option	Sleepy Time Smoothie (p. 157)

LIFESTYLE UPGRADE

Salt can be a huge saboteur of weight loss, causing you to retain water and tipping the scale in the opposite direction you want! And to help along the process of expelling some of the excess water you may already be retaining, there are a couple amazing diuretics you can incorporate into your diet starting today. First, include 5–10 asparagus spears in both your lunch and your dinner. Asparagus's unique mineral profile makes it an effective natural diuretic, promoting the formation of urine in the kidneys and aiding in detoxification and cleansing. Second, drink at least one cup of dandelion root tea, which is popular in not only treating health ailments like digestive disorders, kidney disease, skin irritations, and fever, but it too is a strong natural diuretic that will help flush out your system.

DETOX 101: DO NOT PASS THE SALT

Whether it's a bag of crispy potato chips or a plate of hot, fresh French fries, most of us love a salty treat once in a while. But Americans may not be aware of just how much salt they are actually consuming. Used in many processed foods to bind, add flavor, and preserve, added salt is found in everything from canned soup to pasta sauces, processed meats to canned vegetables, and frozen meals to condiments.

The biggest risk of a high-sodium diet is the effect it has on blood pressure and heart health. Hypertension/high blood pressure, heart disease, and kidney failure are some of the critical health problems that can result from long-term, high-sodium intake. But it can also have an effect on your weight loss efforts as well.

When your diet is too high in salt, the sodium content in your body increases. To offset this increase in sodium, your body begins to retain water, which can translate into a temporary weight gain in the form of "water weight." When you reduce your salt intake, the concentration of sodium declines and the kidneys begin to expel fluids to bring the correct balance of sodium and water in the body. Simply removing added salt from your diet can result in the loss of just over 1 pound of water weight on the first day! After about a week, you may see a loss in water weight of up to 3 pounds. Ready to put down those salty potato chips yet?

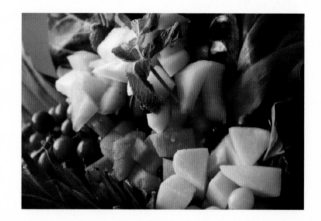

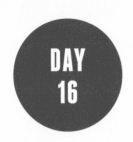

DAY 16

Earlier in this book, we touched on the importance of gratitude in achieving true happiness and peace of mind. But like many things, it takes practice to become a natural, daily occurrence. As you move through your day today, make an effort to pause now and then and think as you do something "I am grateful." I like to do this with my morning cup of tea. Try touching your morning herbal tea with gentle love and appreciation before you take your first sip, grateful for the joy this small practice gives you. Moving through your day with awareness and grace in this way will mean that when you do sit down to write your gratitude list tonight, all the little things you were grateful for today will come to mind.

DAILY AFFIRMATION

"I choose love, joy, and freedom, open my heart and allow wonderful things to flow into my life."

DAILY PREP

Get chopping, get packed, and get organized!

TIP OR TRICK

Suffering from gas or bloating? Try taking a digestive enzyme when you eat (found in your local vitamin and supplement store) and refrain from drinking water while you're eating. Instead, enjoy a big glass of H_2O before your meal.

LIFESTYLE UPGRADE

Modern life is full of hassles, deadlines, frustrations, and demands—all of which lead us to feel totally stressed out. For many people, stress is so commonplace that it has become a way of life, but this can take a major toll on your health. Because of the long-term damage too much stress can cause, it is important to find ways to manage it and allow your mind, body, and spirit to relax on a daily basis. Read this week's Detox 101 to learn a some effective (and simple) techniques to de-stress and restore mental balance.

MORNING CLEANSE DRINK	BREAKFAST	MID-MORNING SNACK	LUNCH	MID-AFTERNOON SNACK	DINNER	EVENING SNACK (OPTIONAL)
Serenity Now Juice (p. 135)	Choose 1 Salad Option	Weight Loss Tonic: Green Juice with Grapefruit (p. 133)	Choose 1 Lunch or Salad Option	½ banana 1 handful natural nuts	Cellulite Crusher Greens Salad (p. 144)	Cooling Nighttime Cucumber Juice (p. 159)

We all get a little stressed out sometimes. From work to social to family obligations, it's easy to get overwhelmed. But stress can wreak havoc on both your health and your weight loss efforts. In fact, stress and excess fat storage go hand in hand, one triggering the other. When you are under stress, your body releases a stress hormone called cortisol from the adrenal glands. Unfortunately, an over secretion of cortisol will lead to weight gain, typically in the abdominal region. It can also slow down metabolism and trigger cravings for junk food.

The long-term activation of the stress-response system—and the subsequent overexposure to cortisol and other stress hormones—can disrupt almost all your body's processes. This puts you at increased risk of numerous health problems including heart disease, sleep problems, digestive problems, and depression.

But there are some simple ways to achieve instant stress relief. Here are some of my favorite tricks:

1. **Use a stress ball**—yep, one of those squishy, kitschy balls. The simple mechanical act of squeezing actually does dampen stress while also massaging some key acupuncture points in the hand.

2. **Inhale some relaxing essential oils.** My trick is to put some lavender oil on a tissue or handkerchief and carry it with me throughout the day.

3. **Have a laugh!** Laughter lowers blood pressure, relaxes your muscles, and can even reduce the levels of stress-creating hormones. Youtube is a go-to of mine for funny videos.

4. **Open up your (third) eye.** The spot in the center of your forehead is known as your "third eye," and massaging it with a little sesame oil has been shown to have a calming effect. Use gentle, circular motions for as long as is comfortable—but the longer, the better.

5. **Knuckle tapping**—known as the "thymus tap," this method of rhythmically tapping your knuckles on your chest has a soothing effect. The beat should follow a pattern of one heavy tap followed by two lighter taps (think of the steps in a waltz: one, two, three. One, two, three). Tap for two minutes.

6. **See blue, not red.** Color therapists suggest that the color blue has a way of lowering stress and blood pressure. A blue light bulb might be hard to come by, so in a pinch simply close your eyes and visualize yourself bathed in blue light. Breathe deeply and picture all the stress floating out of your body as you exhale.

7. **Sigh or yawn widely.** This action releases tension held in the jaw, which is a common stress spot. Groaning loudly can also help.

8. **Sip a glass of water . . . very . . . slowly.** A form a mindful meditation, this simple act can be calming. Be conscious of the water in your mouth, its temperature, and the way it feels going down your throat.

9. **Any form of deep breathing.** Try the Detox Breath I outlined earlier in the program.

10. **Get active!** Jog on the spot, do some jumping jacks, or stretch out your tense muscles. Anything to get those endorphins flowing and release some pent-up energy.

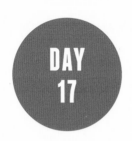

DAY 17

Today I want you to acknowledge a truth that is crucial for you to accept in order to achieve the success you crave: There is no longer any time left for settling. There's no time to say "I will do/have/be that when I get older/retire/save money/make a plan." Your time is now. Go big. Go HUGE. And know that everything and anything you want is yours for the taking. You simply have to want it.

DAILY AFFIRMATION

"Good and positive love is flowing to me and through me at all times."

DAILY PREP

Get chopping, get packed, and get organized!

TIP OR TRICK

Do as the French do! Ever wonder how French women can eat things like butter, pastries and creamy cheese and seem to stay so svelte and stylish? Well, the key is smaller portions! Take a page from their playbook and leave some room in your tummy when enjoying a meal. Eat slowly, allow yourself to enjoy each bite, and when you get the signal you are getting full—put down the fork!

LIFESTYLE UPGRADE

Today's lifestyle upgrade is simple: Make your home as toxin free as possible by performing as many simple tasks as possible from today's Detox 101's Tips for Detoxifying Your Home list. Aim for at least 5, but of course the more changes you can make, the better!

MORNING CLEANSE DRINK	BREAKFAST	MID-MORNING SNACK	LUNCH	MID-AFTERNOON SNACK	DINNER	EVENING SNACK (OPTIONAL)
Cold Fighter Vitamin C to the Rescue! (p. 127)	Weight Loss Tonic: Green Juice with Grapefruit (p. 133)	Bone Builder Juice (p. 132)	Gut Happy Arugula Salad with Lemon Dill Dressing (p. 147)	The Craving Crusher (p. 119)	Amazing Mulligatawny Detox Soup (p. 152)	1 cup chamomile tea 1 cup celery sticks 10 natural almonds

So we've covered how to eliminate internal toxins from our body, but what about the toxins in our homes? The average home contains 500-1,000 chemicals, many of which we are unable to see, smell or, taste. While these chemicals may be tolerated individually and in small doses, problems can arise when we are exposed to them in combination or in larger doses. In fact, the air inside our homes is typically 2–5 times more polluted than outdoor air. Home insulation, although great for keeping our homes warm in winter and cool in summer, doesn't allow fresh air in, so we're constantly breathing in the same stale air. Wall-to-wall carpeting keeps us cozy, but can introduce a myriad of toxins to our well-insulated homes. It can also trap dirt, fleas, dust, dust-mites, and lead. Furthermore, many of the cleaning products we use to clean our furniture, bathrooms, windows and so on are full of toxic chemicals, some of which do not even appear on the labels.

This may make you feel panicky—but don't worry, it is possible to make your home as toxin-free as possible by taking a few simple steps:

1. **No shoes in the house.** Most household dirt, pesticides, and lead are dragged in by wearing your shoes indoors. Take your shoes off immediately upon entering, and go barefoot or wear slippers when at home.

2. **Place floor mats vertically by your entryways to wipe your shoes.** This way more dirt and residue from your shoes stays outside on the mat

3. **Keep the air clean.** Keep your windows and doors open as much as possible to ventilate—at least 15 minutes, twice a day. Use green plants as natural air detoxifiers, remove odors with baking soda instead of chemical-filled room spray, and use fresh flowers or bowls of herbs like rosemary and sage to add a pleasant fragrance to rooms. Have your air ducts and vents cleaned with nontoxic cleaners (there are many organic cleaning companies) and get a portable air cleaner/purifier, especially for the bedrooms.

4. **Switch to cleaner and greener household cleaning products.** They work just as well as standard cleaners, and they don't damage your health or the environment. Even better, make your own natural cleaners using basic ingredients you have around the house. For instance, vinegar in place of bleach, baking soda to scrub your tiles, and hydrogen peroxide to remove stains.

5. **Use plastics wisely** as some contain Bisphenol A (BPA), which is linked to cancer and Phtalates, which are linked to endocrine and developmental problems). Avoid plastic food packaging (when you can), don't wrap food in plastic, and don't microwave food in plastic containers. When choosing products for your children, choose baby bottles made from glass or BPA-free plastic, avoid vinyl teethers for your baby, and stay away from children's toys marked with a "3" or "PVC."

6. **Get a professional to remove toxic waste.** Whether it's removing asbestos from your attic or old lead paint cans from the garage or basement—do not handle these tasks yourself. Let the experts handle these dangerous toxins.

7. **Keep household dust to a minimum.** Mop all surfaces at least once a week and use a vacuum cleaner (with a HEPA filter, preferably) for

your carpets. HEPA-filter vacuums capture the widest range of particles and get rid of allergens.

8. **Avoid excess moisture** as it encourages the growth of mold and mildew. Check areas for moisture accumulation or leaks (particularly basements). Regularly clean surfaces where mold usually grows—around showers and tubs and beneath sinks.

9. **Get a shower filter** (as many of the contaminants in tap water become gases at room temperature). A shower filter can help keep these toxins from becoming airborne.

10. **Get a water filter.** More than 700 chemicals have been identified in drinking water, and filtering your tap water is better than drinking bottled water.

11. **Avoid stain-guarded clothing, furniture, and carpets** (due to the presence of PFCs). Wrinkle-free and permanent press fabrics used for clothing and bedding commonly contain formaldehyde—use untreated fabrics where possible. Also, when you bring dry cleaning home, leave it outside and uncovered for 30 minutes to air out the toxins used in the cleaning process.

12. **Be conscious of toxins in carpeting, especially in products made from synthetic materials.** Choose natural fiber wool and cotton rugs, and if possible, replace your wall-to-wall carpeting with hardwood floors, all natural linoleum, or ceramic tiles. Use nontoxic glues, adhesives, stains, or sealers for installation.

13. **Make your garden and outdoor space organic.** Replace toxic lawn and garden pesticides and herbicides with less harmful natural ones, and use natural compost to grow your flowers and food.

14. **Look for natural, untreated cotton sheets.** Many linens are treated with formaldehyde. Wash new sheets in hot water to remove their finish.

15. **Have your house checked for carbon monoxide leaks,** (most commonly found in leaking gas stoves, gas fireplaces, furnaces and chimneys and gas water heaters). If you have a fireplace, make sure you have it professionally cleaned regularly.

Although it's important to take steps to reduce our risk of chronic illness by limiting our exposure to these toxins, don't let this become an obsession. Too much stress in itself is toxic!

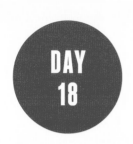

DAY 18

Sometimes when we start a new spiritual path, so many awesome shifts begin to happen that it's easy to become overly enthusiastic about them and want to share every detail with your loved ones. But the new developments in your life may not be easy for people to understand, especially if they're not on a spiritual path of their own. This new lifestyle might even scare people who are forced to look into the mirror and acknowledge that they too could use a little positive change. Be gracious and understanding that although they love you, they may not be able to understand the importance of this journey to you. However, don't let the judgment of others bring you down either. You are doing what's right for you—no apologies required!

DAILY AFFIRMATION

"I am now ready to accept a happy, fulfilling relationship."

DAILY PREP

Get chopping, get packed, and get organized!

TIP OR TRICK

Try making your own trail mix. Throw in some raw unsalted nuts, raisins, dried goji berries, and unsweetened cranberries, and some cacao nibs (for you chocolate lovers). Toss it all together in an airtight container, or, plan ahead and make individual baggies that you can quickly grab when you're on the go.

LIFESTYLE UPGRADE

Take your yoga practice to the next level and try a Kundalini yoga class! Kundalini Yoga is one of the most powerful and effective forms of yoga, working to balance the energy systems in the entire body, including the brain and the glandular and nervous systems. This allows you to function at a consistently higher level, without exhausting your mind and body. And the positive effects can be felt almost instantly! New to yoga? Not a problem. There are classes for beginners too.

MORNING CLEANSE DRINK	BREAKFAST	MID-MORNING SNACK	LUNCH	MID-AFTERNOON SNACK	DINNER	EVENING SNACK (OPTIONAL)
Prego Juice! (p. 136)	Choose 1 Breakfast Option	½ cup plain yogurt mixed with 1 tsp. ground flax	Avocado Salad (p. 147)	Choose 1 Snack Option	Amazing Mulligatawny Detox Soup (p. 152)	Cooling Nighttime Cucumber Juice (p. 159)

This program has taught you how to detox your body, and yesterday we talked about the importance of detoxing your environment. But there is one area left that needs to be detoxed: your personal life. Yes, I'm talking about toxic relationships—those relationships that drain your self-esteem and your energy, and isolate you from your loved ones. Perhaps you have encountered a toxic coworker or family member, or have been involved in a toxic romantic relationship. No matter what the situation is, toxic relationships are harmful for both your mental and physical health, so it's important to recognize when you are involved in one and get help accordingly.

I want you to complete a quick exercise: Start by making a list of the people in your life and place them into three categories. The first is people who affect you positively (make you feel good); the second is people who affect you negatively (make you feel bad); and the people who have no real effect on you. Take time to contemplate who these people are to you and how much time you invest in each one. I'd be willing to bet the people who are in the "make you feel bad" category demand the most from you, robbing you of the time you could be spending with the people who make you feel good.

So now you have two choices: you can either abandon the negative relationships entirely; or change them. This can be a tough choice, especially when the negative people are family members or people whom you are bound to in some way (such as children) and therefore less easily discarded.

Here are some ways you can decide if you are in a toxic relationship that you need to remove yourself from and how to successfully do it:

1. **Don't ignore a gut feeling.**

We often know something is wrong far earlier than we care to admit. Start paying attention to your reactions to negative people and situations involving them. How does your body react in any given moment? Are you fearful? Do you recoil? That's your body giving you some important information.

2. **Don't let your past cloud your judgment.**

We all have our own individual filters, which impact how we act in our relationships today and what we perceive as being "healthy" or "unhealthy." For example, if you grew up in an environment where one parent constantly belittled the other, and you find yourself in a similar situation, it may not raise as big a red flag for you as it should. The challenge becomes filtering all of your past influences to recognize the difference between gut feelings and simply interpreting events based on fear or past experiences.

3. Don't place blame on yourself.

Be cautious of selling yourself short. The aggressors in a toxic relationship will often play on your fears and weaknesses as a way to manipulate or control. It is common to place the blame on ourselves and engage in negative self-talk, such as "I'm not relationship material" or "I'm never going to find anyone else." By doing so, we end up settling or staying in a relationship that is unhealthy because we are fearful of what life would be like without it.

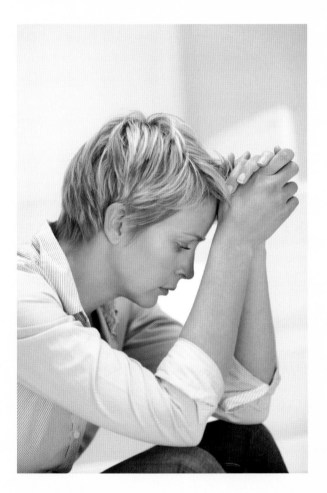

4. Remove yourself from the relationship.

As hard as it may be, making the decision to remove yourself from a toxic relationship is imperative to your emotional and mental well-being. Since this can be daunting, you need to take baby steps and not be afraid to ask for help from a professional or close, trusted friend or family member.

Once you've managed to remove yourself from a toxic relationship, you must begin reshaping and rebuilding of your self-esteem from the inside out to ensure you don't find yourself in a similar situation in the future. Additionally, shift your focus to spending more quality time with family, friends, and coworkers who support you and make you feel good.

You are an important and worthy individual who deserves only love and positivity. Surrounding yourself with people who reinforce this truth is the best way to achieve a truly toxic-free life!

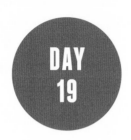

DAY 19

By now most people have heard of "The Secret," a movement based on the idea that your thinking dictates what you attract in your life. Thus, if you think negatively, you will attract negative things into your life, and vice versa. "The Secret" might only have come about in the last decade, but spiritual gurus have been preaching this for centuries. And it's a truly empowering way of thinking, because it gives you control over what happens in your life. Today I want you to ask the universe for what you desire most. Picture it in your head and believe that it is yours to have. Do this each and every day until your belief becomes reality!

DAILY AFFIRMATION

"I enjoy performing small acts of kindness for those I love, including myself."

DAILY PREP

Get chopping, get packed, and get organized!

TIP OR TRICK

Taking a vacay or work trip? Don't let that become an excuse to leave your new active lifestyle at home. There are plenty of ways to sneak in some physical activity. The easiest one is to walk everywhere you can! For example, skip the train in the airport and walk through the concourses instead. If you feel up for a light jog instead, go for it! People are used to seeing sprinters in the airport so don't worry about stares from strangers. When you reach your destination, rent a bike to get about town instead of driving. Or take the stairs in your hotel instead of the elevator. Simple things like this add up quickly!

MORNING CLEANSE DRINK	BREAKFAST	MID-MORNING SNACK	LUNCH	MID-AFTERNOON SNACK	DINNER	EVENING SNACK (OPTIONAL)
Fertility Juice (p. 136)	Choose 1 Juice Option	1 brown rice cake topped with 1 tsp. natural nut butter and ground cinnamon	Beet, Avocado, and Kelp Salad (p. 143)	½ red apple 1 cup baby carrots and sliced fennel	Choose 1 Dinner or Entree Option	Cooling Nighttime Cucumber Juice (p. 159)

LIFESTYLE UPGRADE

Apples! They say just one of these babies a day keeps the doctor away; but did you know that it also helps to keep you looking great? The secret is in their skin, which alone provides 2–6 times the antioxidant power of the rest of the apple. What's more, just one large apple has 5.7 grams of fiber, which is great for cleansing and making sure your digestive system is functioning properly to help you maximize weight loss and keep your appetite at bay. Plus, they are extremely portable and easily tossed in your purse. So enjoy a juicy apple daily and keep the doctor and the pounds away!

DETOX 101: MOOD SWINGS AND PMS

Most of us have had those days where we seem to be riding a rollercoaster of emotion—going from happy to irritable in the blink of an eye. Often this is a reaction to a biochemical change when our blood sugar levels drop. And for many the instant reaction is to reach for a chocolate bar or some other sweet treat to cope.

However, this is not a healthy solution to dealing with mood swings. Instead we need to address what imbalances are causing them and deal with them in a more positive way. And we can do this by changing what we put in our bodies. For example, if you are prone to drops in blood sugar that lead to irritability, try reaching for a banana instead of a cookie.

Alcohol is another factor that contributes greatly to our mental state. Too much alcohol depletes the liver's B vitamins, which are responsible for maintaining a good state of mind.

Coffee is another big culprit for mood swings because of the caffeine. Try switching to decaf herbal teas instead.

Women in particular often suffer from emotional ups and downs during their menstrual cycle. A good fix for these mood swings are symptom-reducing herbal teas and some methods of relaxation, such as deep breathing exercises. Chaste berry and skullcap teas can balance hormones and relieve other physical symptoms, such as tension. Feverfew eases headache pain and can start your menstruation flow if it needs a little assistance. And guelder rose, aptly nicknamed "cramp bark," is used to relieve premenstrual cramps. Just make sure that any herbal teas you drink are decaffeinated, as caffeine can aggravate PMS symptoms. I have also provided a delicious recipe for a PMS relief smoothie! You can find it in the recipe section of the program.

Once you realize the foods or drugs that are contributing to your mood swings, taking back control by cutting down or cutting them out completely is simple. Changing what you put into your body is a long-term solution to a more balanced and happier you!

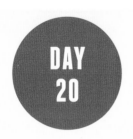

DAY 20

You are nearing the end, my friend. Are you excited? Nervous? Hopeful? Take some time today and write it all down—your hopes for the future; what challenges you want to take on next; areas where you can continue to grow. The finish line is in sight—don't give up until you've triumphantly crossed it!

DAILY AFFIRMATION

"I continue to climb higher and higher. There are no limits to the heights I can reach."

DAILY PREP

Get chopping, get packed, and get organized!

TIP OR TRICK

Napoleon Hill is famous for saying, "Whatever you conceive and believe, you can achieve." Ain't that the truth! The universe absolutely, positively, undeniable supports you in anything you believe. You were created entitled to infinite abundance. But we often lose that belief. We start to believe that getting a job/making money/losing weight is supposed to be hard. That we're supposed to struggle. That it's normal. Well, I'm here to remind you that it's not. It's as easy as believing that you not only deserve it, but it's yours to reach out and take! So go ahead, reach out, and take it.

LIFESTYLE UPGRADE

Get arts and craftsy and create a vision board. What the heck is a vision board? Typically it's simply a poster board on which you paste or collage images that you've torn out from various magazines or printed from the web that inspire or represent the positive things you want in your life. The idea behind this is that when you surround yourself with images of who you want to become, what you want to have, where you want to live, or where you want to vacation, your life changes to match those images and those desires. And now that you're approaching the end of this journey, what better time to create a clear vision of what you want moving forward? Just try not to over think it. This exercise is about feeling your way through it. When finished, place it somewhere where it will inspire you daily!

MORNING CLEANSE DRINK	BREAKFAST	MID-MORNING SNACK	LUNCH	MID-AFTERNOON SNACK	DINNER	EVENING SNACK (OPTIONAL)
The Metabolism Shocker (p. 133)	Choose 1 Breakfast Option	Workout Wonder Juice (p. 128)	Choose 1 Salad Option	½ cup plain yogurt mixed with 2 Tbsp. natural granola	Choose 1 Salad Option	Sleepy Time Smoothie (p. 157)

CONSTIPATION AND "HEALTHY POO"

BMs, doo-doo, poop—whatever you want to call it, we all know what it is and we all do it (hopefully) every day. But despite our familiarity with the action itself, most people don't truly understand its importance and its role in their gastrointestinal health.

Bowel movements are important for your health because they are the body's natural way of excreting waste from the body. Although many people have questions about their bowel movements and what a proper one is, there is no real "normal" when it comes to frequency, color, shape, and size. The general rule of thumb is that normal bowel movements are defined as what's comfortable for you. However, being knowledgeable about your digestive process can help you identify when normal goes awry.

Frequency: When it comes to frequency of bowel movements, there's no real normal, only averages. The average is once or twice a day, but some people go more and some people go less. If you are comfortable, you don't need to over think it.

Color: Bowel movements are generally brown in color because of bile, which is produced in the liver and important to the digestion process. It typically takes three days from the time you eat your food until the time you pass it. If it takes a shorter time, the result may be greener stool because green is one of the first colors in the rainbow of the digestive process.

Paying attention to color is important, since it is often a sign that something is wrong. For example, stool that is black can mean that you are bleeding internally, possibly as a result of an ulcer or cancer. However, black stools are common when taking a vitamin that contains iron or medications that contain bismuth subsalicylate, so be aware of the effects of any supplements you are taking on your stool.

Stool that is light in color, like grey clay, can also mean trouble if it's a change from what you normally see. Although uncommon, very light-colored stool can indicate a block in the flow of bile or liver disease.

Size and shape: Size used to be used as an indication of a problem, but not anymore. In reality, size is irrelevant.

Odor: Some people like to think theirs doesn't stink, but in truth it is normal if your poop does! In fact, it's most likely a good sign that your gut is abundant with bacteria that is working hard to keep you healthy. Furthermore, your intestines are swarming with trillions upon trillions of bacteria that enhance digestive and metabolic processes, and their presence is also the reason why poop smells. So if yours doesn't smell like roses, that's normal!

Constipation: *Constipation is unfortunately a common concern for many. You can consider yourself constipated when you normally have a bowel movement once or twice a day, and that changes, perhaps going three days, or more. However long it's been, you feel gassy, bloated, and generally uncomfortable.*

Constipation can be caused by many things, including a shift in your diet, such as a drop in fiber intake, not drinking enough water, or a drop in your physical activity that slows down your metabolic processes, including digestion. Certain medications (such as narcotic pain medicines and iron supplements) can also cause constipation.

If this is a common problem for you, try eating some foods that have natural laxative effects, like bananas, apples, berries, avocados, and nuts. You can also try herbal teas such as dandelion root or chickweed, which are both considered mild herbs with laxative action. Also, opt for whole grains regularly and eat lots of fresh fruits and vegetables that are high in fiber and whose vitamins and minerals will help keep your digestive system working at its best. Flax seeds are also a great way to keep things moving. Sprinkle ground flax on your oatmeal, your salads, or include them in a smoothie.

Generally, you recoup from a bout of constipation in a day or two. If the problem persists, it's probably worth a trip to the doctor for further investigation.

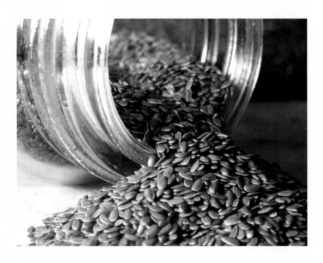

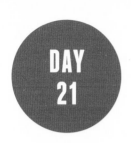

DAY 21

You made it! How do you feel? Is your hair shining? Is your mind buzzing with positive energy and clarity? Is your body feeling toned and healthy? I'm guessing the answer is a resounding "YES!" to all of these questions. You are a powerful being. Be so proud of making it to the end of this detox adventure, and be excited about beginning the next chapter in your new, healthier life.

DAILY AFFIRMATION

"I am the embodiment of success and am becoming better every day."

DAILY PREP

Get chopping, get packed, and get organized!

TIP OR TRICK

Still not 100% confident in yourself and your ability to conquer the world? Well, as the saying goes: Fake it 'til you make it! Much like the placebo effect of the medical world, studies show that simply acting out a certain belief can manifest it into a reality. Therefore, acting like you're confident and happy can actually make you confident and happy. You are amazing and deserve a joyous life. Act out this truth each and every day, and in no time you will be projecting your awesomeness to the world with true conviction and without apology!

LIFESTYLE UPGRADE

I hope that over the last 21 days you have kept your eye on the prize, each day revisiting the goals and action plan you set on Day 2 of this journey. Now it's time to create a new action plan and new goals to carry forward into the rest of your new and improved life! This is a great time to challenge yourself even further now that you've laid the foundation for a healthier lifestyle and mental well-being. Don't be afraid to push yourself outside your comfort zone—success is yours if you want it badly enough! Believe and you can achieve.

MORNING CLEANSE DRINK	BREAKFAST	MID-MORNING SNACK	LUNCH	MID-AFTERNOON SNACK	DINNER	EVENING SNACK (OPTIONAL)
Citrus Wheatgrass Juice (p. 125)	Choose 1 Breakfast Option	Choose 1 Juice Option	Choose 1 Salad Option	1 brown rice cake topped with 1 tsp. natural nut butter and ground cinnamon	Choose 1 Salad or Entree Option	1 cup chamomile tea 1 cup celery sticks

You have made it to the end of your journey, making it more important than ever to stay focused and keep moving toward the happier and healthier life you committed to on Day 1. This means continuing to build on the momentum you've created so far.

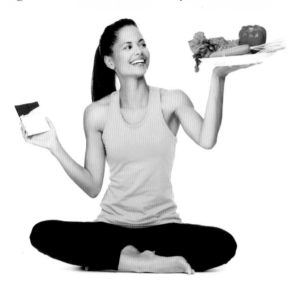

Change involves overcoming certain roadblocks, including bad habits, self-sabotage, and unforeseeable challenges. But only by continuing to move forward do we ever reach our destination.

There are many negative emotions that can impede our progress toward a more happy and healthy life. Negative emotions communicate to your body that there is some form of threat out there—that in some way you are not safe. But you can eliminate negative emotions by getting to the source of these feelings.

After all, our emotions don't develop out of nowhere; we create them.

More specifically, it is our beliefs that create our emotions. For example, one simple dysfunctional belief, such as "everyone hates me," can generate a plethora of negative emotions that will plague someone daily. On the other hand, a more positive belief, such as "I'm safe and loved," can make someone happy and content for an entire lifetime.

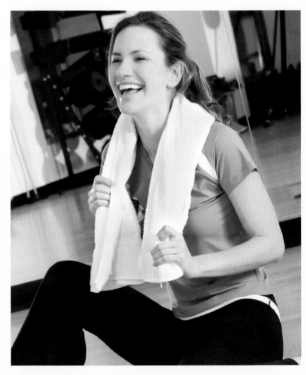

When you change your beliefs, you instantly and permanently transform your emotional state. Let's look at an example as it applies to weight loss: Imagine that you have arbitrarily decided at some conscious or subconscious level that being overweight is in some way making you safer. By holding this belief, you will continually undermine your efforts no matter how hard you struggle to lose weight. If you were to change your thinking so that instead you believed that the thinner you are, the safer you are, your weight problems would be solved.

One simple thought, one simple change, and weight loss becomes almost effortless. Keep this in mind moving forward as this 21-day journey ends and the rest of your life begins.

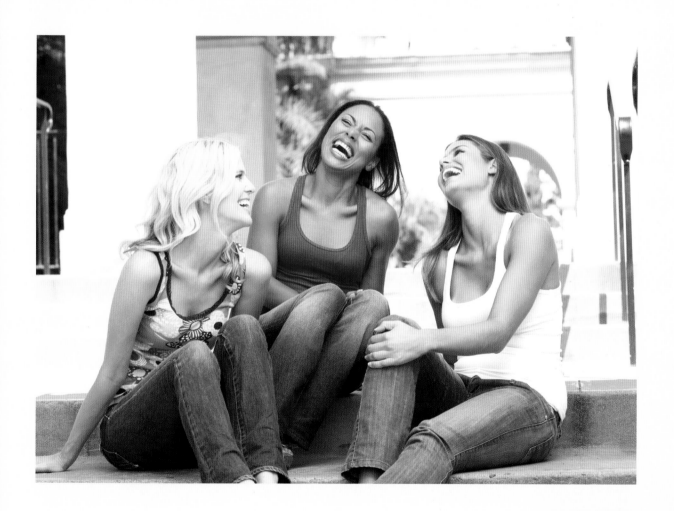

CONCLUSION
CONGRATULATIONS ON COMPLETING THIS AMAZING JOURNEY OF DETOXIFICATION!

Be proud of yourself and what you have accomplished in the last 21 days—I certainly am! And remember, just because this journey is over doesn't mean I'm no longer here for you. I hope you join me online where the conversation is always flowing!

I am a big fan feedback and hearing personal experiences, so don't be a stranger.

Your partner in change,

Adele Cavaliere

Ready for your next challenge? *Sign up for my 7 Day Juice Detox—a fantastic juicing journey that will take your health to the next level by extensively cleansing your body of toxins, boosting your immune system, banishing cravings, increasing your energy, and slimming your waistline. Visit www.adelefridman.com for more information.*

RECISPE

RECIPES

SMOOTHIES

Rise and Shine Shake

Protein is an important component of any meal, but it is particularly important when it comes to breakfast. This yummy shake offers a good dose of protein to start the day, along with important omega-3 fats. So wake, shake, and go!

1 tsp. coconut oil/butter

1 Tbsp. ground or whole hempseeds

1 cup papaya, fresh or frozen

1 Tbsp. cacao nibs

1 Tbsp. bee pollen granules

1 cup unsweetened plain almond or hemp milk

1 scoop iso—whey- or plant-based protein powder, your choice of flavor

water + ice for added thickness

COMBINE all ingredients in your blender and blend until smooth. Pour and enjoy!

PMS Relief Shake

Vitamin B can be a girl's best friend, and the almonds and yogurt in this thick and delicious smoothie are chock-full of them! Enjoy the yummy flavor and the relief from PMS symptoms including bloating, cravings, tiredness, and mood swings.

1 cup fresh or frozen strawberries

½ cup fresh or frozen raspberries

10 natural almonds, preferably soaked overnight

1 tsp. organic dark honey

1 tsp. magnesium powder

1 tsp. glutamine powder

½ cup plain Greek yogurt

water + ice for added thickness

COMBINE all ingredients in your blender and blend until smooth. Pour and enjoy!

Thyroid Support Shake

The lauric acid found in coconut oil stimulates thyroid function, increasing metabolism and weight loss, while the iodine found in spirulina and sea salt supports both thyroid gland and brain function. Kick-start your weight loss with this sweet and salty thyroid-rousing smoothie!

1½ cups unsweetened plain almond or hemp milk

1 cup fresh or frozen strawberries

½ cup cooked millet or ½ cup instant plain rolled oats

1 tsp. spirulina

1 scoop iso—whey- or plant-based protein powder, your choice of flavor

1 tsp. kelp or Celtic sea salt

1 tsp. bee pollen granules

1 tsp. coconut oil/butter

water + ice for added thickness

> **COMBINE** all ingredients in your blender and blend until smooth. Pour and enjoy!

Get in the "Mood" Smoothie!

Romance or chocolate? It's best to have both! Dark chocolate contains a chemical known as phenylethylamine that stimulates the sense of excitement and well-being. Pumpkin seeds are high in zinc, which is essential for healthy reproduction and preventing testosterone deficiency in men. They are also loaded with libido vitamins and minerals like vitamins B, E, C, D, K, and minerals including calcium, potassium, niacin, and phosphorous. So go ahead and get romantic with this "exciting" smoothie!

1 cup fresh or frozen blackberries, blueberries, or strawberries

1 tsp. ground flax seeds

½ cup instant plain rolled oats

1 scoop chocolate iso—whey- or plant-based protein powder

⅓ cup natural pumpkin seeds

⅓ avocado

1 Tbsp. grated dark chocolate or ⅓ cup cacao nibs

2 tsp. maca root powder

1 cup unsweetened plain almond or hemp milk

water + ice for added thickness

> **COMBINE** all ingredients in your blender and blend until smooth. Pour and enjoy!

Sweet Bee Pollen Smoothie

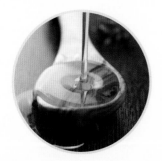

Bee pollen contains all the nutrients needed to sustain life, which is why it is being used on an ever-larger scale for human nourishment and health. Bee pollen works wonders in a weight-control or weight-stabilization regimen by correcting a possible chemical imbalance in body metabolism that may be involved in either abnormal weight gain or loss. Enjoy the normalizing and stabilizing effects of this perfect food from the bees in this sweet smoothie treat!

1 cup unsweetened plain almond or coconut milk

1 Tbsp. bee pollen granules

1 tsp. organic dark honey

1 Tbsp. natural nut butter

1 scoop chocolate iso—whey- or plant-based protein powder

1 cup fresh or frozen strawberries

1 tsp. matcha green tea powder

½ cup instant plain rolled oats

water + ice for added thickness

COMBINE all ingredients in your blender and blend until smooth. Pour and enjoy!

Go Bananas Protein Shake

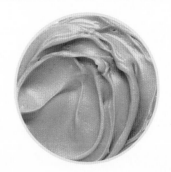

Protein, protein, and more protein! Between the almond milk, nut butter, chia seeds, and protein powder, this deliciously frothy smoothie will rev your metabolism and keep you full for hours! Go nuts, go bananas, and go blend one now!

1 cup unsweetened plain almond or coconut milk

1 Tbsp. natural nut butter

1 Tbsp. chia seeds

1 tsp. ground organic cinnamon

½ vanilla bean (can substitute with 1 tsp. pure vanilla extract if unavailable)

1 scoop vanilla iso—whey- or plant-based protein powder

½ frozen or fresh banana

water + ice for added thickness

COMBINE all ingredients in your blender and blend until smooth. Pour and enjoy!

OMG-3 Smoothie

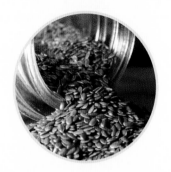

Not only does this smoothie offer a healthy dose of omega-3 from the creamy avocado, but the vitamin K and the iron in the kale helps protect you from many cancers and gives you abundant energy, while the ginger gets that metabolism going! An o-mega delicious combo.

1 handful baby kale

1 handful baby spinach

1 handful parsley

1 tsp. ground flax seeds

1 tsp. ground or whole hemp seeds

10 natural walnuts

1 cup fresh or frozen strawberries

¼-inch piece ginger, peeled

⅓ avocado

water + ice for added thickness

COMBINE all ingredients in your blender and blend until smooth. Pour and enjoy!

Hormone Balance Smoothie

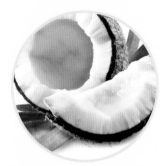

You may think you've died and gone to heaven when you sip this decadently flavored drink! Filled with antioxidants, protein, and a good dose of amino acids, it's the perfect way to "indulge" while stabilizing those hormones.

1½ cups unsweetened plain coconut milk

1 scoop vanilla iso—whey- or plant-based protein powder

1 tsp. organic dark honey

1 cup fresh or frozen raspberries or blueberries

1 tsp. ground flax seeds or hemp seeds

1 tsp. pure vanilla extract

1 tsp. maca root powder

COMBINE all ingredients in your blender and blend until smooth. Pour and enjoy!

Anti-Aging Lime-Coconut Smoothie

The powerful antioxidants found in the amazing matcha green tea powder help combat the free radicals that cannot only cause cancer, but also wreak havoc on your skin. Nuts have also been shown to slow down the clock while also offering a good source of vitamins and minerals, including potassium, which helps lower blood pressure; vitamin E, which helps prevent cell damage (including your skin cells!); and calcium to maintain strong bones. Turn back the clock with this island-inspired drink!

1 cup water

½ cup coconut water

½ avocado

1 lime, juiced

1 small frozen or fresh banana

10 natural almonds, preferably soaked overnight

1 tsp. matcha green tea powder

1 Tbsp. coconut butter/oil

1 Tbsp. coconut flakes

1 tsp. glutamine powder

> **COMBINE** all ingredients in your blender and blend until smooth. Pour and enjoy!

High-Energy Protein Smoothie

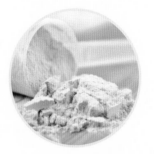

Both brewer's yeast and spirulina are superfoods, offering a plethora of benefits including boosting the immune system, rebuilding blood cells, improving gastrointestinal health, and balancing the microflora in the gut. Combined them with the protein punch of the nut butter, yogurt, and protein powder, this smoothie is a recipe for strong muscles and soaring energy!

1 scoop iso—whey- or plant-based protein powder, your choice of flavor

1 tsp. spirulina

1 tsp. matcha green tea powder

1 cup fresh or frozen strawberries

1 tsp. black strip molasses

1 Tbsp. brewer's yeast

1 Tbsp. natural nut butter

½ cup instant plain rolled oats

1 tsp. glutamine powder

1 cup organic plain yogurt

1½ cups water

> **COMBINE** all ingredients in your blender and blend until smooth. Pour and enjoy!

Calcium Smoothie

We all know the role calcium plays in strong bones and preventing osteoporosis, but studies show that it can also keep you slim! Research suggests calcium may prevent weight gain by promoting more fat to be burned and less fat to be stored. So incinerate that unwanted fat with this delicious, calcium-rich smoothie!

½ cup pre-boiled turnip greens

1 tsp. black strip molasses

⅓ cup natural sesame seeds

2-3 kalamata figs

⅓ cup natural almonds

½ scoop iso—whey- or plant-based protein, your choice of flavor

1 cup unsweetened plain almond or hemp milk

> **COMBINE** all ingredients in your blender and blend until smooth. Pour and enjoy!

Potassium Smoothie

Potassium is involved in nerve function, muscle control, and blood pressure. And because potassium helps build muscle, helps our muscles work properly, and helps us convert the food we eat into energy, it is particularly important to those looking to achieve weight loss. Luckily this smoothie is chock-full of it!

1 small fresh or frozen banana

4 dried, unsweetened apricots

1 cup plain organic yogurt

1 Tbsp. natural pumpkin seeds

1 cup unsweetened plain almond or hemp milk

water + ice for extra thickness

> **COMBINE** all ingredients in your blender and blend until smooth. Pour and enjoy!

Heartburn Eliminator Smoothie

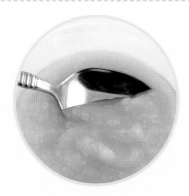

Rolled oats are the perfect food for those suffering from heartburn, since it helps absorb the acidity in your gut and in other foods. Ginger is another great food for acid reflux and has been used throughout history as an anti-inflammatory and as a treatment for gastrointestinal conditions. Combine a soothing cup of ginger tea with this oatmeal based smoothie, and the only thing that will be burning is your metabolism!

1 cup instant plain rolled oats

2 cups unsweetened apple sauce

1 cup coconut water

⅓ cup fresh or frozen blueberries

1 tsp. ground cinnamon

> **COMBINE** all ingredients in your blender and blend until smooth. Pour and enjoy! Enjoy with a cup of gingerp tea.

The Craving Crusher

This naturally sweet treat will help you stop those sugar cravings in their tracks while offering a powerful punch of vitamins and minerals. Deliciously un-sinful!

1 cup unsweetened plain almond or hemp milk

½ cup fresh or frozen strawberries or blueberries

1 Tbsp. ground cinnamon

1 scoop chocolate iso—whey- or plant-based protein powder

1 Tbsp. fresh, chopped mint

½ cup baby spinach

1 tsp. stevia

1 Tbsp. cocao nibs

1 tsp. matcha green tea powder

1 Tbsp. brewer's yeast

water + ice for added thickness

> **COMBINE** all ingredients in your blender and blend until smooth. Pour and enjoy! Enjoy with 1 cup hot chai tea.

Cherry Vanilla Sundae Smoothie

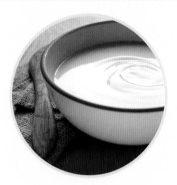

Still craving the white stuff? This smoothie packs a protein punch that will balance your blood sugar levels (thus helping to stomp out your cravings!), while the natural sweetness of the cherries mixed with the always fabulous vanilla will tantalize your taste buds. A smooth, creamy treat!

1 cup water

1½ cups fresh or frozen cherries

1 cup plain Greek or goat yogurt

1 Tbsp. natural almond butter

1 Tbsp. cocao nibs

1 scoop vanilla iso—whey- or plant-based protein powder

1 tsp. pure vanilla extract

1 tsp. ground cinnamon

> **COMBINE** the first 7 ingredients in your blender and blend until smooth. Pour and top with the ground cinnamon. Enjoy!

Estrogen Smoothie

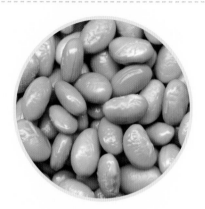

By consuming 50–100 mg of isoflavones (the plant estrogen found in soy products) a day, you can reduce your hot flashes and night sweats, help stop your PMS symptoms, and start to have healthier skin, hair, and nails. The brewer's yeast is high in chromium, helping to lower glucose levels and stimulate immune function. We're feeling cooler already!

1 cup organic unsweetened plain soy milk

½ cup edamame beans, pre-soaked

1 cup fresh or frozen strawberries

⅓ cup ground wheat germ

1 scoop iso—whey- or plant-based protein powder, your choice of flavor

1 tsp. black strip molasses

1 tsp. brewer's yeast

water + ice for added thickness

> **COMBINE** all ingredients in your blender and blend until smooth. Pour and enjoy!

Homemade Muesli

If you are looking for a high-energy, whole-grain food that will also help you get your daily dose of healthy fats and soluble fiber and fuel your for the day ahead, then look no further! This Muesli recipe uses four grains, as well as some dried fruit and nuts and seeds, to make a very flavorful cereal.

1 cup medium or thick plain quick rolled oats or oat flakes

½ cup rolled rye flakes

½ cup rolled wheat flakes

½ cup dried unsweetened dates

⅓ cup natural walnuts or pecans, chopped

¼ cup ground flax seeds or flaxseed meal

¼ cup natural sesame seeds

⅓ cup dried unsweetened goji berries

MIX the ingredients together in a large bowl. Transfer to an airtight container. If storing for longer periods, consider keeping the cereal in the freezer or refrigerator.

Hot Muesli Instructions:

ADD ½ cup Muesli to ½ cup water or unsweetened almond milk and bring to a boil. Simmer for 3–5 minutes. You can also microwave Muesli in a large bowl on high for 3–5 minutes, stirring once halfway through.

Cold Muesli Instructions:

SOAK ¼ cup Muesli in ½ cup yogurt for 5–10 minutes, or soak overnight.

Cholesterol Buster Muesli Breakfast

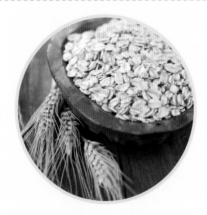

½ cup medium or thick plain quick rolled oats

½ cup rolled barley flakes

½ cup slivered almonds

⅓ cup dried unsweetened raisins

1 tsp. coconut butter/oil or 1 Tbsp. coconut flakes

1 tsp. ground flax seeds

½ cup dried unsweetened mango or papaya

⅓ cup natural chopped macadamia nuts

⅓ cup dried unsweetened prunes

MIX the ingredients together in a large bowl. Transfer to an airtight container. If storing for longer periods, consider keeping the cereal in the freezer or refrigerator.

SERVE either hot or cold (as per instructions for Homemade Muesli recipe on previous page), with chopped fresh banana or green apple.

Nut "ella" Lovers' Breakfast Porridge

Nuts, nuts, and more nuts! This recipe for nut fanatics uses sliced almonds, pecans, walnuts, and pistachios to give you a daily dose of healthy fats, omega-3 fatty acids, and powerful antioxidants that can help you recover after a hard workout.

½ cup medium or thick plain quick rolled oats

½ cup rolled barley flakes

¼ cup natural slivered almonds

¼ cup natural chopped walnuts

½ scoop chocolate iso—whey- or plant-based protein powder

⅓ cup ground wheat germ

¼ cup natural chopped pecans

¼ cup natural hazelnuts

1 Tbsp. hazelnut chocolate spread

MIX the ingredients together in a large bowl. Transfer to an airtight container. If storing for longer periods, consider keeping the cereal in the freezer or refrigerator. Serve either hot or cold.

HOT INSTRUCTIONS: Add ½ cup porridge to ½ cup water or unsweetened almond milk and bring to a boil. Simmer for 3–5 minutes.

COLD INSTRUCTIONS: Soak ¼ cup porridge in ½ cup yogurt or unsweetened almond milk for 5–10 minutes, or soak overnight.

Lean Muscle Fruit 'n' Protein Pancakes

Looking for a breakfast or snack that's not only delicious, but bread-free? Look no further! These protein-filled pancakes will stave off the bread cravings while giving you a dose of metabolism revving protein with a side of spice! Research shows that lean muscle helps burn fat at rest—so this muscle packing breakfast is the perfect start to get into your summer clothes!

¼ cup liquid free-run egg whites

1 scoop vanilla iso—whey- or plant-based protein powder

2 Tbsp. unsweetened plain almond or hemp milk

1 tsp. cinnamon

1 Tbsp. ground flaxseed

¼ cup plain instant rolled oats

⅓ banana, mashed

1 Tbsp. plain Greek yogurt

1 Tbsp. natural coconut flakes

¼ cup fresh blueberries, mashed

1 tsp. organic dark honey

1 tsp. grape seed oil

COMBINE first 6 ingredients and mix. Mix in the mashed banana, followed by the yogurt, berries, and honey. Heat pan on medium heat and add oil. Pour batter into the pan and leave until you see little bubbles forming on top. Flip and then cook until the middle is done. Serve and enjoy!

Sweet Cherry Almond Oatmeal

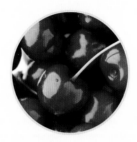

Unlike regular quick oats, steel cut oats haven't be processed and therefore haven't been stripped of a lot of their vitamins and minerals. This recipe combines the goodness of the oats with some of my favorite spices, the sweetness of cherries, and the crunch of almonds. It's a warm, stick-to-your-gut way to start the day!

½ cup steel cut oatmeal

¼ cup ground flaxseed

1 tsp. ground cinnamon

¼ tsp. Celtic sea salt or kelp

1 tsp. pure vanilla extract

1 Tbsp. natural nut butter

4 cups water

½ cup unsweetened dried fruit (cherries, goji, or cranberries)

10 natural almonds

BRING water to a boil in a saucepan. Stir in the first 6 ingredients, reduce heat, and simmer for 20–30 minutes. Once oats have reached desired consistency, remove from heat and stir in cherries and almonds. Ladle into bowls and enjoy!

Berry French Toast (makes 2 slices)

This protein-packed French toast is a sure fire way to fill your tummy and quell those sugar cravings! Makes an excellent breakfast, but can also be a great snack too!

1 whole egg

3 liquid free-run egg whites

¼ cup unsweetened plain almond milk with a dash of spice—cinnamon and/or nutmeg

2 slices spelt, gluten-free, or yeast-free toast

¼ cup fresh blueberries

1 tsp. coconut butter/oil

1 Tbsp. unsweetened coconut flakes

1 tsp. organic dark honey

BEAT egg and egg whites, milk, and spices together. Heat griddle or non-stick pan over medium heat and add the coconut butter to the pan. Dip bread in egg mixture, place on griddle, and cook for 3 minutes on one side. Flip and cook for one more minute until egg is cooked through. Top toast with berries, coconut flakes, and honey. Serve and enjoy!

Protein-Packed Asparagus Omelette

This omelette features asparagus, which is nutrient-dense and flavorful while containing no fat, no cholesterol, and low sodium, making it an ideal candidate to round out any meal. One of the higher protein vegetables, asparagus has an amino acid, asparagine, named after it! And since it's a natural diuretic, it prevents the water retention that leads to water weight. Ready to crack some eggs yet?

¼ cup liquid free-run egg whites

1 whole egg

1 handful baby kale

4 cherry tomatoes, sliced

4 broccoli florets, sliced

4 asparagus spears, sliced

1 tsp. grape seed oil

1 tsp. ground flax seeds

1 red grapefruit, squeezed

COMBINE the first 6 ingredients together in a large mixing bowl. Heat frying pan with oil on medium heat. Add liquid mixture. Flip when mixture seems to pack. Top with ground flaxseed and serve. Enjoy with the fresh-squeezed grapefruit juice.

WHEATGRASS JUICES

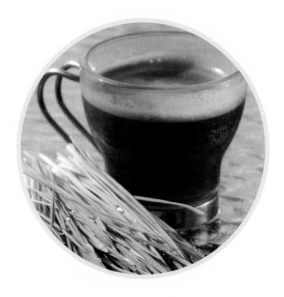

Wheat grass really is a superfood. It increases red blood-cell count and lowers blood pressure. It cleanses the blood, organs, and gastrointestinal tract of debris, while aiding in the reduction of blood pressure by dilating the blood pathways through-out the body. It also stimulates metabolism and the body's enzyme systems by enriching the blood. And as if all that wasn't enough, it also restores alkalinity to the blood. Juicing it is a great and easy way to reap all of its benefits. Here are some excellent wheatgrass juice combos:

Citrus Wheatgrass Juice

2 oranges

1 Tbsp. fresh, grated ginger

30 ml. wheatgrass juice

RUN first 2 ingredients through your juicer and mix in wheatgrass juice. Pour and enjoy!

Green Apple Wheatgrass Juice

3 large carrots

2 green apples

2 ribs celery

1 Tbsp. fresh, grated ginger

30 ml. wheatgrass juice

RUN first 4 ingredients through your juicer and mix in wheatgrass juice. Pour and enjoy!

Punchy Purple Wheatgrass Juice

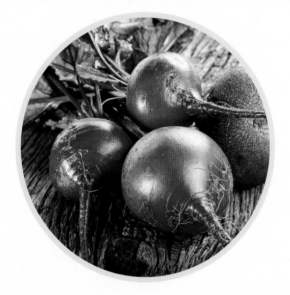

2 medium cucumbers

½ beetroot

2 ribs celery

30 ml. wheatgrass juice

> **RUN** first 3 ingredients through your juicer and mix in wheatgrass juice. Pour and enjoy!

Zesty Lemon Wheatgrass Juice

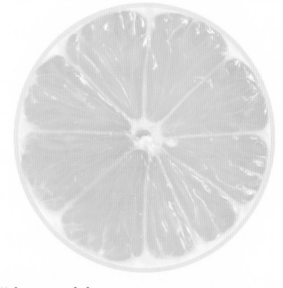

½ lemon, peeled

1 handful of fresh parsley

1 handful of fresh mint

30 ml. wheatgrass juice

> **RUN** first 3 ingredients through your juicer and mix in wheatgrass juice. Pour and enjoy!

Minty Breath Wheatgrass Juice

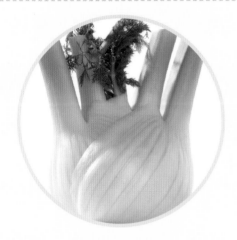

2 ribs celery

2 ribs fennel

1 handful of fresh mint

30 ml. wheatgrass juice

RUN first 3 ingredients through your juicer and mix in wheatgrass juice. Pour and enjoy!

Cold Fighter Vitamin C to the Rescue!

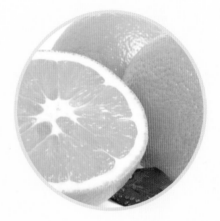

The combination of these veggies and fruits offer a large dose of vitamin C, allowing you to absorb iron and beta-carotene, which converts to vitamin A in the body, helping you to produce collagen and boost your immune system. No one wants a spring cold—so drink up!

1 orange

2 large carrots

1 green apple

1 clove garlic

¼-inch piece fresh ginger

1 tsp. organic dark honey

RUN first 5 ingredients through your juicer. Pour, add honey, and mix with a spoon. Enjoy!

Tummy Warming Tonic

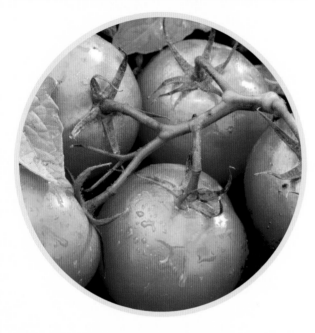

With the thermogenic properties of ginger on its side, this juice is warm in both color and effect. Chase away the winter chill with this deliciously spiced veggie cocktail!

2–3 medium vine-ripe tomatoes

1 large carrot

2 ribs fennel

2 ribs celery

1-inch piece fresh ginger

1 clove garlic (optional)

> **RUN** all ingredients through your juicer, pour, and enjoy!

Workout Wonder Juice

The natural sugars in this vitamin packed green juice will give you the kick you need to get the most out of any workout. Plus, the anti-inflammatory properties of the kale and the spinach will help you avoid injury. Drink up and get moving!

½ pear, cored

½ green apple, cored

2 ribs celery

½ grapefruit

½ lemon, peeled

2 cups baby kale or collards (veins removed)

1 cup baby spinach

¼-inch fresh ginger

1 tsp. ground cinnamon

1 tsp. ground turmeric

1 tsp. glutamine powder

> **RUN** first 8 ingredients through your juicer and pour. Feel free to add water if you find the consistency too thick. Add cinnamon, turmeric, and glutamine to your finished juice, mix with a spoon, and enjoy!

We Got the "Beet" Juice

Recognized for their awesomely vibrant color, beets are a great boost to your physical well-being and a wonderful source of iron. They have also been shown to be an immunity booster and guard against cancer. When combined with these other glorious green veggies, it's a recipe for detox deliciousness!

2 large golden or red beets

1 large cucumber

3 ribs celery

2 cups baby kale

2 cups romaine lettuce

1 lime, peeled

> **RUN** all ingredients through your juicer, pour, and enjoy!

Refreshing Cucumber Basil Juice

Cabbage looks ordinary enough, but it's full of vitamin C and fiber, and has been used to effectively treat constipation, stomach ulcers, excess weight, heart disease, aging, and Alzheimer's disease. Combine it with the classic combination of cucumber and basil and you have a wonderfully fresh and nutrient-rich cocktail!

1 cup cabbage

1 cup fennel

½ large cucumber

½-inch piece pineapple, sliced

¼ cup fresh basil

¼-inch piece fresh ginger

½ medium green apple, cored

> **RUN** all ingredients through your juicer, pour, and enjoy! If desired, add 1 teaspoon of manuka honey and a squeeze of lemon for added taste and mix with a spoon.

A Forest of Fiber Juice

Spinach AND swiss chard—so much fiber! Combined with iron packed watercress, this juice is simple yet nutrient packed. Go green and get juicing!

2 cups romaine lettuce

2 cups baby spinach

4 watercress leaves

4 swiss chard leaves, deveined

1 grapefruit, peeled

> **RUN** all ingredients through your juicer, pour, and enjoy!

Belly Bloat Beating Juice

Get all the thermogenic benefits of delicious ginger, combined with the sweetness of sweet potato and cinnamon. A spiced treat to fire up any metabolism!

1 small sweet potato, unpeeled

2 medium carrots

1 large red or orange bell pepper

2 large ribs celery

¼-inch fresh ginger

¼ tsp. ground cinnamon

¼ tsp. ground turmeric

¼ tsp. ground nutmeg

> **RUN** first 5 ingredients through your juicer and pour.

> **STIR** in spices and enjoy!

Red and Tangy Goddess Juice

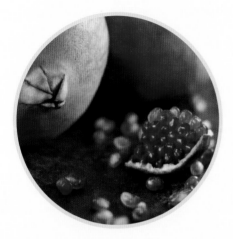

The Greek goddess Persephone loved pomegranates, and so should you! Not only are they yummy, but they are filled with heart-healthy antioxidants called punicalagins. Combine it with the detoxing qualities of kale and the anti-inflammatory properties of ginger, and you've got a drink good enough for the gods!

1½ cups baby kale

1 cup pomegranate arils

1 cup fresh cranberries

½ pear, cored

¼-inch piece fresh ginger

6–12 leaves fresh mint

> **RUN** all ingredients through your juicer, pour, and enjoy!

Renewing Juice

Defy aging with this delicious juice! Tomatoes offer a dose of lycopene, which has been shown to smooth skin and even protect it from harmful UV rays, while the vitamin C found in lemons stimulates collagen production, helping to prevent fine lines.

1 large cucumber

1 large hothouse tomato

1 rib celery

½ avocado

1 tsp. ground turmeric

1 rib fennel

½ lemon, peeled

> **RUN** all ingredients through a juicer, pour, and enjoy! If desired, add 1 teaspoon glutamine powder to your finished juice and mix with a spoon.

"Get Glowing" Skin

Water Retention Juice

The combination of asparagus and dandelion root makes this juice a natural diuretic powerhouse. Combined with the tummy filling fiber of the apple, this juice will have you slimming down in no time!

8 asparagus spears

2 ribs celery

2 large dandelion root leaves

1 cup cilantro

¼–inch piece fresh ginger

½ large cucumber

1 small lemon, peeled

½ green apple, cored

> **RUN** all ingredients through a juicer, pour, and enjoy! Enjoy with a cup of hot milk thistle tea.

Bone Builder Juice

Collard greens, spinach, and kale are filled with calcium, and just one cup of collard greens gives you 800% of your daily vitamin K requirements, another nutrient vital in building strong bones. So forget milk—whip up this amazing bone-building juice!

½ pear, cored

1 small green apple, cored

3 apricots, cored

1 orange, peeled

1 cup baby spinach

1 cup collard greens

2 cups baby kale

> **RUN** all ingredients through a juicer, pour, and enjoy!

Weight Loss Tonic: Green Juice with Grapefruit

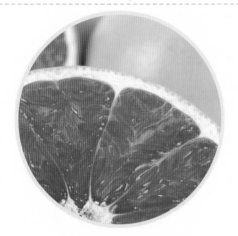

This combination of ginger, grapefruit, and pectin is a fantastic weight loss tonic. Grapefruit is low in calories but high in fiber, so it makes you feel fuller without packing on the pounds. Ginger lowers cholesterol, increases metabolism, and improves gastric mobility. And finally, pectin stabilizes insulin and blood sugar levels while also providing a good dose of fiber. A rockstar trio for weight loss!

½ small green apple

1 grapefruit, peeled

1 rib celery

1 head of romaine lettuce

¼-inch piece fresh ginger

1 medium cucumber

1 lime, peeled

> **RUN** all ingredients through your juicer, pour, and enjoy!

The Metabolism Shocker! Celery-Apple-Kiwi with Turmeric Juice

The high content of dietary fiber in the kiwi and the apple helps control blood sugar levels, while spicy turmeric helps limit fat expansion in the body so you can eat more without storing so much fat! Shock your metabolism into fat burning mode with this sweet and spicy juice.

2 ribs celery

1 small red apple

1 kiwi

⅓ cup fresh parsley

1 Tbsp. ground turmeric

> **RUN** first 4 ingredients through your juicer and pour. Stir in turmeric and enjoy!

Bikini Body Fruit Juice

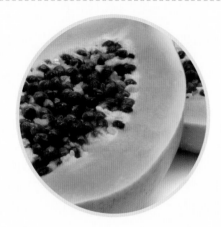

Called "the fruit of the angels" by Christopher Columbus, papaya is rich in antioxidants and fiber, helping you both slim down and fight disease. Blueberries have been shown to reduce abdominal fat while lowering cholesterol. Combine these fruits with the others, which are rich in beta-carotene—the essential ingredient to healthy hair, clear eyes, and healthy skin—and you've got the perfect recipe for looking gorgeous on any beach!

1 orange, peeled

1 cup fresh papaya, peeled and seeded

2 1-inch thick slices pineapple

2 1-inch thick slices watermelon, peeled and seeded

1 cup fresh blueberries

> **RUN** all ingredients through a juicer, pour, and enjoy! If desired, add 1 teaspoon glutamine powder to your finished juice and mix with spoon.

Cardio Apple and Beet Juice

Beets are not only fat free, they are also a strong diuretic that flush out floating body fats. And at only 88 calories for 2 beets, these deliciously vibrant vegetables are a great food for maintaining your fat loss! Furthermore, a recent study has shown beets to improve cardio endurance by replenishing oxygen stores during your workout! Blend this juice up for an amazing pre-workout snack.

2 red beets

1 small red apple, cored

1 cup baby spinach

1 rib celery

1 lemon, peeled

> **RUN** all ingredients through a juicer, pour, and enjoy!

Muscle-Building Spinach Juice

Oh spinach—where do I even start? Spinach is full of fiber, which leaves you feeling fuller for longer, while also improving your digestive system and lowering your cholesterol. It's also rich in selenium that will keep your metabolism humming steadily, burning energy and aiding weight loss. Plus, it's high in protein, helping you build lean, strong muscles! Hey, it's good enough for Popeye! Note: Juice cucumbers with their skins on. The dark green skin is a great source of chlorophyll, a phytochemical that can help build red blood cells.

1 cup baby spinach

1 large cucumber

2 ribs celery

2 large carrots

1 small green apple

> **RUN** all ingredients through a juicer, pour, and enjoy! If desired, add 1 tablespoon ground brewer's yeast to your finished juice and mix with a spoon.

Serenity Now Juice

If you're looking for calm and serene, look no further than the flavors in this deliciously simple juice. A sweet and mellow concoction—perfect for a relaxing weekend afternoon.

½ cup papaya

1 orange

½ mango

> **RUN** all ingredients through your juicer, pour, and enjoy!

Prego Juice!

Pears are not only deliciously sweet, but they also contain vitamins A, C, K, B2, B3, and B6. Important for expectant or nursing moms, they also contain folate. Pears aren't too shabby in the mineral department either, containing calcium, magnesium, potassium, copper, and manganese. Vitamin C and copper are antioxidant nutrients, so eating pears is good for your immune system and may help prevent cancer. Pears also contain boron, which our bodies need in order to retain calcium, so this fruit can also be linked to osteoporosis prevention. Phew—need we say more?

2 Bartlett pears

1 medium green apple

1 red bell pepper

2 large carrots

1 tsp. bee pollen granules

> **RUN** first 4 ingredients through your juicer and pour. Add bee pollen to your finished juice and mix with a spoon. Enjoy!

Fertility Juice

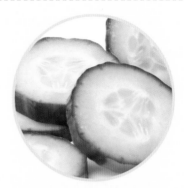

Basil is a pregnancy super food. This fresh herb is a good source of protein, vitamin E, riboflavin, and niacin; plus, it's a very good source of dietary fiber, vitamin A, vitamin C, vitamin K, vitamin B6, magnesium, phosphorus, potassium, zinc, copper and manganese. Basil is also packed with iron, vital for keeping your energy levels up; calcium, essential for strong bones and teeth; and folate, vital for many processes, including fetal cell growth and division. Whenever possible, choose fresh basil, because it contains more of these nutrients than dried.

1 large cucumber

1 medium hothouse tomato

2 large carrots

1 bunch of fresh parsley

1 bunch of fresh basil

1 tsp. black strip molasses

> **RUN** first 5 ingredients through your juicer and pour. Add molasses to your finished juice and mix with a spoon. Enjoy!

Protein-Packed Energy Balls

From the protein powder, to the seeds and nuts, to the nut butter—these protein-packed balls are a perfect treat to get your metabolism fired up! Have them as an appetizer style breakfast or pop a few in your purse as a great on-the-go snack. With these amazing balls around, you'll never reach for a Timbit again!

½ cup natural nut butter

1 scoop chocolate iso—whey- or plant-based protein powder

1 tsp. matcha green tea powder

2 cups instant plain rolled oats

1 tsp. pure vanilla extract

1 tsp. ground cinnamon

1 tsp. ground nutmeg

⅓ cup unsweetened raisins

⅓ cup unsweetened goji berries, finely chopped

1 cup natural coconut flakes

½ cup natural pumpkin seeds

½ cup natural pecans or walnuts

¾ cup cacao nibs

IN a large bowl, mix together the nut butter, protein powder, and matcha green tea powder. Once they are mixed well, fold in the oats, followed by the vanilla, cinnamon, and nutmeg. Next, add the remaining ingredients. Once mixed, roll the mixture in your hands to form 1-inch balls. If your mixture is too dry, you can add some organic honey to the mix. When finished, place balls in an airtight container and place them in the fridge to set. Once set, serve and enjoy!

Flat Tummy Kefir and Yogurt Oat Parfait

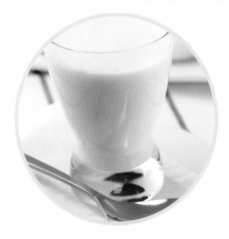

Kefir and yogurt are the ultimate "probiotic" partners in health. Kefir can best be described as a sort of liquid, sparkling yogurt, with its own distinct and deliciously mild, naturally sweet, yet tangy flavor. Honour a balanced gut with this delicious snack that combines these two probiotic powerhouses.

½ cup plain kefir

½ cup plain Greek or goat yogurt

1 Tbsp. chia seeds or salba

2 Tbsp. unsweetened raisins

¼ cup quick plain rolled oats

1 Tbsp. natural shredded coconut

1 tsp. organic dark honey

> **COMBINE** the first 6 ingredients in a bowl. Drizzle with the honey and serve. Delish!

Chia and Tahini Pudding

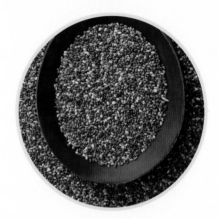

Not only are chia seeds gluten-free, but they are an amazing source of protein (boasting all 8 essential amino acids!), omega-3 fats, calcium, and iron. They also have a positive impact balancing blood glucose levels, which makes them great for weight loss. This sweet and savory pudding is the perfect way to enjoy all of their awesome benefits!

1½ cups water

½ cup tahini (ground sesame seeds)

½ cup chia seeds

1 Tbsp. natural coconut flakes

½ cup crushed blueberries

1 tsp. organic hazelnut spread (optional)

> **PLACE** water in a large bowl or cup and add tahini and chia seeds. Stir until well combined. Let mixture sit for about 10 minutes. Mix in coconut flakes, blueberries, and hazelnut spread (if using) just before serving. Serve and enjoy!

Black Bean Brownies

Looking for a way to sneak some extra fiber into your favorite chocolate treat? Well look no further. Black beans are rich in dietary fiber, helping to control rises in blood sugar and keeping you fuller for longer. They are also high in protein and can increase your energy by helping to replenish your iron stores. In fact, one cup of black beans contains 20% of your daily requirements of this important mineral. These brownies are a dessert you can feel good about!

2 cups cooked black beans, drained and rinsed

1 small fresh banana

⅓ cup black strip molasses

¼ cup natural cacao nibs

1 Tbsp. ground cinnamon

1 tsp. pure vanilla extract

1 tsp. organic dark honey

1 scoop chocolate iso—whey- or plant-based protein powder

¼ cup instant plain rolled oats

PREHEAT oven to 350°F. Grease an 8 × 8 pan and set aside. Combine all ingredients, except oats, in a food processor or blender and blend until smooth, scrapping sides as needed. Stir in the oats. If too soft, add another ¼ cup oats or flour. Pour batter into the pan. Bake for 30 minutes or until a toothpick inserted in the center comes out clean. Allow to cool before slicing. Serve and enjoy!

Very Berry Pudding

This raw dessert boasts a plethora of health benefits. Blueberries help lower cholesterol while also fighting the dreaded abdominal fat, ginger has strong thermogenic properties that boost your metabolism, and avocados give you a dose of heart-healthy omega-3s! This nutrient-rich dessert is not your childhood pudding cup!

1 cup fresh or frozen blueberries

⅓ avocado

3 Tbsp. fresh lemon juice

1 tsp. freshly grated ginger

5 Tbsp. coconut water

3 drops liquid stevia or 1 packet stevia

1 tsp. organic dark honey

COMBINE all ingredients in blender and blend well until mixture is smooth and creamy. Serve immediately as frozen blueberries will thaw and change the consistency of the pudding.

Sweet Potato Pie Pudding

Looking for something that tastes like your favorite holiday dessert but offers up an abundance of vitamins and minerals instead of an expanding waistline? You got it!

1 medium sweet potato, baked, peeled

1 scoop vanilla iso—whey- or plant-based protein powder

pinch of Celtic sea salt

½ tsp. ground nutmeg

½ tsp. ground cinnamon

½ tsp. ground pumpkin spice

1 Tbsp. natural walnuts, chopped

BLEND the first 6 ingredients in your blender until smooth yet thick in consistency. Spoon into a bowl and sprinkle with walnuts. Yum yum!

SALADS

Cucumber Salad with Mint

The fresh spearmint adds a unique flavor dimension to this nutrient packed salad. Between the immune-boosting vitamin C in the bell pepper; the omega-3s in the avocado; and the iron and calcium in the dark greens—this salad packs a detoxifying punch zested up with the fresh lime. Toss and enjoy!

2 large cucumbers, chopped

⅓ avocado, chopped

½ orange bell pepper, chopped

1 cup baby spinach

1 cup baby kale

1 bunch spearmint

1 lime, squeezed

1 Tbsp. balsamic vinegar

1 tsp. Celtic sea salt

IN a large bowl, combine cucumber, avocado, and bell pepper. Dice spinach, kale, and spearmint and add to bowl. Squeeze lime, drizzle vinegar, and sprinkle salt over top of the salad. Mix well, serve, and enjoy!

Vitamin D Kale and Portobello Mushroom Salad

Nicknamed the "sunshine vitamin," vitamin D not only promotes mental well-being, it also plays an important role in helping your body absorb calcium, promoting the maintenance of healthy bones and teeth. Fortunately, heart-healthy tuna is high in this important vitamin, making this salad an excellent source. Soak up the sunshine (vitamin) by tossing up this delicious salad.

1½ cups baby kale

2 large Portobello mushrooms, sliced

5 cherry tomatoes

½ (3-oz) tin low-sodium Skipjack tuna

1 Tbsp. pressed goat cheese (optional)

2 Tbsp. balsamic vinegar

IN a large bowl, combine kale, mushrooms, tomatoes, and tuna. Crumble goat cheese over the mix and drizzle with vinegar. Toss, serve, and enjoy!

Sweet Potato Lentil Salad

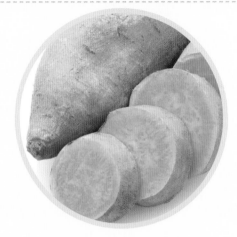

Sweet potatoes are a slow-digesting carb, making them great for weight loss. They have a copious amount of fiber, which makes a happy digestive system, and their sweet flavor actually helps fight sugar cravings. Furthermore, their beta-carotene is converted to vitamin A in the body, a powerful antioxidant that helps fight the signs of aging. Regular potatoes just can't beat these vibrant health superstars!

½ sweet potato, cut into chunks or fries

½ tsp. extra-virgin olive oil

½ tsp. ground cinnamon

2 cups arugula salad

½ (3-oz.) tin low-sodium white tuna

2 Tbsp. cooked green lentils

4 cherry tomatoes

2 Tbsp. balsamic vinegar

PREHEAT oven to 400 °F. Place sweet potatoes on a baking sheet and drizzle with oil and sprinkled with cinnamon. Toss to coat then transfer to oven. Bake for 20 minutes or until tender. Remove and let cool slightly.In a large bowl, combine arugula, tuna, lentils, and tomatoes. Add the sweet potatoes. Drizzle with vinegar and toss well. Serve and enjoy!

Beet, Avocado, and Kelp Salad

Beets are not only bright in color, but they are also bright in flavor and offer high levels of anti-carcinogens and carotenoids, which are powerful antioxidants that can help prevent some forms of cancer and heart disease, and act to enhance your immune response to infections. Kelp contains many vitamins, especially B vitamins, which are essential for cellular metabolism and providing your body with energy. It also contains vitamins C and E, which are both strong antioxidants and promote blood vessel health. Avocado oil provides a healthy dose of omega-3 and is fantastic for skin health. So slim down and get glowing skin with this yummy salad!

3–5 kelp seaweed strips

1 small cucumber, chopped

1 small beet root, peeled

½ green apple, cored and diced

⅓ cup fresh dill, minced

½ lemon, juiced

2 Tbsp. avocado oil

1 Tbsp. apple cider vinegar

¼ tsp. Celtic sea salt

½ avocado, sliced

PLACE kelp in a large bowl or pan and cover with filtered water. Set aside and let soak for 20 minutes.

IN a food processor or blender, blend cucumber, beet, and apple until combined but still a little chunky. Drain and rinse seaweed and cut into thin strips. In a small bowl, whisk together dill, lemon juice, oil, vinegar, and salt. Transfer the beet mixture into a large bowl and add kelp strips. Pour dressing over the mixture and toss well. Plate the salad and top with avocado. Serve and enjoy!

Cellulite Crusher Green Salad

Hydrated skin appears less dimpled because the more water there is in your skin cells, the plumper the skin will be over the fat boxes and the less the dimpling will show. Healthy fats, like the ones found in flaxseed and avocado, hydrate the skin because they encourage fluid to remain inside the skin cells rather than in the fat cells. Losing overall body fat can also aid in the elimination of cellulite. Apple cider vinegar helps by balancing your blood sugar levels and preventing fat storage. So beat those pesky dimples with this delicious green salad!

2 cups arugula salad

½ avocado, diced

¼ cup fresh blueberries

½ cup sprouts, such as alfalfa

½ cup pineapple, cut into chunks

1 tsp. ground flaxseed

1 tsp. avocado oil (olive oil works if unavailable)

1 Tbsp. apple cider or balsamic vinegar

2 Tbsp. fresh grapefruit, squeezed

> **OPTION:** to make this a heartier salad, add 3–4 ounces of grilled or baked chicken, turkey breast, white fish, or salmon.

> **COMBINE** first five ingredients in a large bowl and sprinkle the flaxseed on top. In a small bowl, whisk together oil, vinegar, and grapefruit juice. Pour over salad mixture and toss well. Plate and enjoy! If using chicken, turkey, or fish, simply lay over top of the plated salad.

Fiber-full Berry Chicken Salad

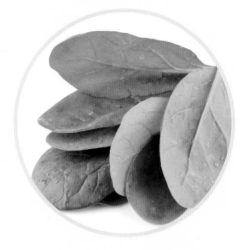

This hearty salad is chock-full of fiber, and is filling enough for lunch or dinner! Toss and enjoy!

2–3 cups baby spinach

3 oz. grilled skinless chicken or turkey breast

¼ cup fresh raspberries or strawberries

2 Tbsp. natural walnuts or almonds, chopped

2 Tbsp. grapefruit juice, freshly squeezed

1 tsp. extra-virgin olive oil or grape seed oil

1 Tbsp. apple cider vinegar

> **COMBINE** first 5 ingredients in a large bowl. In a small bowl, whisk together oil and vinegar and pour over the mixture. Toss and enjoy!

Heart Booster Pomegranate Salad

This alkaline salad is rich in vitamins and minerals. Fennel not only boasts a delicious licorice flavor, but is also a rich source of vitamin C and manganese, as well as loads of alkaline minerals such as calcium and phosphorus. Carrots contain huge amounts of beta-carotene (good for your eyes!), and vibrant pomegranate is an alkaline powerhouse, with its strong antioxidant properties that neutralize free radicals. Furthermore, pomegranates are great for your heart, helping to prevent hardening in your arteries and leading to better blood flow to your heart, and your muscles! Enjoy this quick and healthy salad as a main or side dish.

1 pomegranate

3 Tbsp. fresh lemon juice

5 Tbsp. fresh grapefruit juice

1 Tbsp. extra-virgin olive oil

1½ cup carrots, grated

1 fennel bulb, cut into strips

2 Tbsp. water

sea salt

CUT pomegranate in half and scoop out flesh and seeds. In bowl, mix 1½ tablespoons lemon juice, grapefruit juice, and oil. Add pomegranate and carrots and mix well. In a separate bowl, mix fennel with remaining lemon juice, water, and a little sea salt. Combine all ingredients in one large bowl and toss well. Plate and enjoy!

OPTIONAL: To make this a heartier salad, add 4 ounces of lean protein such as grass-fed beef, salmon, chicken breast, turkey breast, or halibut.

Walnut, Fig, and Lentil Detox Salad

Part of the human diet since neo-lithic times, lentils offer an array of benefits, including a high iron content, five B-vitamins, potassium, and zinc. And with only 115 calories per cup, lentils are low-calorie but high in soluble fiber, meaning they fill you up, help you stay full, and stabilize your blood sugar! An excellent choice for detoxers, particularly those who are vegetarian or vegan.

1½ cups cooked brown lentils, cooled and drained

1 cup baby kale

6 kalamata figs

¼ cup natural walnuts, chopped

1 Tbsp. extra-virgin olive oil

1 Tbsp. balsamic vinegar

2 tsp. organic dark honey

1 Tbsp. Dijon mustard

1 Tbsp. fresh rosemary, chopped

1 clove garlic, crushed

½ tsp. Celtic sea salt

IN a large bowl, toss the lentils, kale, figs, and walnuts together and set aside. In a small mixing bowl, whisk together oil, vinegar, honey, mustard, rosemary, garlic, and salt. Pour over the lentil mix and toss until well combined. Allow to sit at room temperature for at least 20 minutes, allowing the flavors to come together. Stir well before serving. If you want to enjoy as a cold salad, you can refrigerate in an airtight container for at least an hour before serving.

My Good Greens Salad

We've already discussed all the amazing health benefits of spinach, but arugula also offers its share of vitamins and minerals. Arugula contains about eight times the calcium, five times the vitamin A, vitamin C and vitamin K, and four times the iron as the same amount of iceberg lettuce. Although leafy, it's actually classified as a cruciferous vegetable, which are especially useful in protecting against certain cancers. Combine it with monounsaturated fat-packed sesame seeds, which keep your heart healthy and aid digestion, and you've got a green salad that will definitely do your body good.

2 cups arugula

1 cup baby spinach

⅓ avocado, sliced

½ green bell pepper, sliced

2 mini cucumbers, chopped

1 tsp. flaxseed oil

2 Tbsp. balsamic vinegar

⅓ cup fresh lemon juice

¼ cup fresh lime juice

1 Tbsp. natural sesame seeds

IN a large bowl, toss together arugula, spinach, avocado, bell pepper, and cucumber. In a small bowl, whisk together oil, vinegar, lemon juice, and lime juice. Pour over salad mixture and toss well. Sprinkle in sesame seeds, serve, and enjoy!

OPTIONAL: To make this a heartier meal, add 4 ounces of lean protein, such as grass-fed beef, salmon, chicken breast, turkey breast, or halibut.

Gut-Happy Arugula Salad with Lemon Dill Dressing

Omega-3s, which are plentiful in both the avocado and the cashews in this salad, are crucial in maintaining proper gastrointestinal function, keeping your gut happy and healthy! You'll also get a good dose of iron and calcium from all the dark, leafy greens, and an immune-boosting dose of vitamin C from the lemon juice. So full of flavor, this salad will keep your gut and your taste buds happy!

1½ cups arugula

1 cup baby kale

1 cooked yellow beet, grated

4 baby carrots, chopped

½ orange bell pepper, sliced

½ avocado, sliced

1 cup alfalfa sprouts

½ cup natural cashews, chopped

½ cup lemon juice

1 tsp. Dijon mustard

10 fresh basil leaves, chopped

10 fresh dill stems, chopped

1 tsp. avocado oil

1 tsp. Celtic sea salt

1 tsp. organic dark honey

IN a large bowl, combine arugula, kale, beets, carrots, peppers, avocado, sprouts, and cashews. In a small bowl, whisk together lemon juice, Dijon, basil, dill, oil, sea salt, and honey. Pour over salad mixture and toss well.

Avocado Salad

We love avocados for the delicious flavor and creamy texture they add to salads, but they do so much more than please our palate. Avocados have proven cancer fighting abilities due to a certain toxin they contain that is able to kill and prevent the growth of cancer cells. Furthermore, potassium in avocados can regulate blood pressure, while their oleic acid can help lower cholesterol. Delicious and cancer fighting? Yes, please!

2 medium avocados, sliced

2 Tbsp. fresh lime juice

4 oz. radishes, thinly sliced

1 large red bell pepper, chopped

5–6 oz. alfalfa sprouts

1 clove garlic, minced

4 Tbsp. extra-virgin olive oil

1 Tbsp. fresh basil, chopped

pepper and sea salt to taste

IN a large bowl, add avocado and sprinkle with some of the fresh lime juice. Add radishes, pepper, and sprouts. In a small bowl, whisk together garlic, oil, remaining lime juice, basil, and salt and pepper. Pour the dressing over the vegetables and toss well. Serve and enjoy!

"Baby got Brains" Maple-Glazed Walnut-Crusted Salmon

Walnuts have been coined "brain food" not only because they look like a brain (two bumpy off-white lobes), but also because of their ability to aid in proper brain function. Our brains are composed of 60 percent structural fat, and in order to function properly this structural fat needs to be primarily composed of omega-3s, which is found in abundance in walnuts. Salmon is also an amazing source of omega-3 fats, making this dish truly brain food!

1 Tbsp. grape seed oil

4 oz. wild salmon

⅓ cup natural walnuts, crushed

1 Tbsp. natural maple syrup

⅓ cup lemon juice

1 handful fresh, minced dill

2 cups steamed bok-choy

PREHEAT oven to 350°F. Coat a large baking tray with the grape seed oil. Add salmon to the coated tray. Top salmon with crushed walnuts and maple syrup. Bake for 20–25 minutes, or until flaky. Top with lemon juice and dill and serve with steamed bok-choy on the side. Enjoy!

Chunky Beef Stew (2 servings)

Real beef, that is to say grass-fed beef, is a bona fide health food. It's packed with high-quality protein, omega-3s, and even conjugated linoleic acid (CLA). It's also low in the things that you need less of: saturated fat and omega-6s. Corn-fed meat can become loaded with pro-inflammatory omega-6s and saturated fat, and the anti-inflammatory omega-3s are practically nonexistent. Warm up with a bowl of this heart-healthy stew!

½ lb. boneless grass-fed beef (chuck, shank), trimmed of visible fat and cut into 1-inch cubes

2 Tbsp. organic tomato paste

5 cherry tomatoes

2 Tbsp. balsamic vinegar

1 large yellow or white onion, chopped

1 yellow bell pepper, chopped

½ cup white mushrooms, chopped

2 large carrots, chopped

½ sweet potato, chopped

2 fresh cloves garlic, chopped

1 dried bay leaf

1 tsp. dried thyme

1 tsp. ground coriander

1 cup water

1 Tbsp. extra-virgin olive oil

2 tsp. Celtic sea salt

PREHEAT oven to 350°F. Chop veggies and meat. Brown meat cubes in olive oil in a large oven-safe pot with a lid. Next, add remaining ingredients and bring to a simmer. Once simmering, carefully remove from heat and transfer the oven-safe pot to the oven and cook for 2–2½ hours or until meat is tender. Remove bay leaf before serving. Ladle into bowls and enjoy!

Detox-Style Green Chili (2 servings)

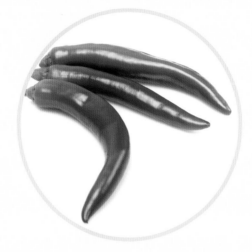

As mentioned before, grass-fed beef provides a good dose of omega-3s, which have been shown to improve the flow of blood to the muscles during exercise and help to promote the enzymes that burn fat for energy. Furthermore, animals raised on feedlots (as opposed to naturally raised) are given diets to boost productivity and lower costs. Although they are fed genetically modified grain and soy, they may also get stale pastry, chicken feathers, and candy . . . even the wrappers. Stick with the grain-fed beef found in this detox chili and stay toxin- (and wrapper-) free!

4 oz. ground grass-fed beef

2 large white onions, chopped

4 cloves of fresh garlic, chopped

1 Tbsp. extra-virgin olive oil

5 cups diced green chilies, roasted, peeled, and finely diced

3 cups organic low-sodium beef, vegetable, chicken, or turkey stock

1 Tbsp. ground coriander

1 Tbsp. ground thyme

IN a large pot, brown ground beef. Next, in a pan, sauté onions and garlic in olive oil and add to cooked ground beef. Add green chilies and stock. Simmer for 1–2 hours. Serve with gluten-free tortillas or blue corn tortilla chips. If desired, top with sliced avocado and chopped cherry tomatoes for extra flavor. Serve and enjoy!

Lean Muscle-Building Bison Burger

One of my favorite protein sources, naturally-raised bison is not only delicious, but offers a host of vitamins, such as iron, which aids in many metabolic reactions and the regulation of cell growth and differentiation. It also encourages the proper function of the liver, an important detox organ! So get grillin' and detox with this awesome bison burger.

1 oz. goat cheese, crumbled

⅓ cup sun-dried tomatoes, drained and chopped

2 cloves garlic, chopped

1 Tbsp. ground cumin

salt and pepper to taste

1 lb. ground naturally-raised (grass-fed) bison

gluten-free pitas

1 bunch arugula

1 hothouse tomato, sliced

1 oz. prepared mustard

COMBINE cheese, sun-dried tomatoes, garlic, and spices in a bowl. Add bison and lightly mix the ingredients together. Form the meat into even-sized patties. Place burgers on a preheated grill and cook for about 4 minutes per side over medium heat, or until an internal temperature of 160°F is reached. Serve on gluten-free pita and garnish with the arugula, sliced tomato, and prepared mustard.

Amazing Mulligatawny Detox Soup

Get whisked away to eastern lands with this delicious soup that not only features my top 3 must-eat spices, but is also vegan! So please, get your soup on!

1 tsp. extra-virgin olive oil

4 cloves fresh garlic, minced

1-inch piece fresh ginger, peeled and grated

2 tsp. ground curry powder

1 tsp. ground turmeric

½ tsp. ground cayenne pepper

1 medium sweet onion, peeled and diced

4 medium carrots, peeled and diced

1 cup cauliflower florets, chopped

1 large Granny Smith apple, cored, peeled, and diced

2 cups cabbage, thinly shredded

6 cups water

1 (16-oz.) can chickpeas, drained and rinsed

small pinch of Celtic sea salt, to taste

2 cups unsweetened coconut milk

juice from 1 lime
(tip: rolling a room temperature fruit across a hard surface will loosen its juices!)

chopped fresh cilantro for garnish

HEAT the olive oil over medium high heat. Add the garlic, ginger, curry, turmeric, and cayenne and stir until fragrant, about 30 seconds. Add the onion, carrots, cauliflower, apple, and cabbage, and sauté until softened, 7–10 minutes. Stir in the water, chickpeas, and sea salt. Bring to a boil and reduce heat, cover, and simmer, stirring occasionally, until vegetables are tender, 20–30 minutes. Remove from heat and add the coconut milk and lime juice. Stir to combine. Return to the heat on low (do not let it come to a boil as the coconut milk will curdle). Adjust seasoning as required. Ladle into bowls and enjoy!

Superfood Quinoa Pasta

Quinoa is a true power food. It is a complete source of protein and has a healthy dose of dietary fiber, an important factor in slowing digestion and slimming your waistline! Furthermore, its magnesium content has been shown to help migraine sufferers due to its relaxing effect on blood vessels. It's also extremely versatile, making a great breakfast porridge in place of traditional oatmeal, an excellent side dish to protein, or as a warm or hot salad on its own—as this delicious recipe demonstrates!

8 oz. fresh artichoke hearts

2 Tbsp. extra-virgin olive oil

1 cup quinoa

5 oz. fresh roma tomatoes, chopped

1 clove garlic, minced

1 tsp. yeast-free vegetable stock

3 Tbsp. fresh basil, chopped

2 Tbsp. fresh mint leaves, chopped

1 pinch cayenne pepper

½ tsp. organic sea salt

PREPARE fresh artichoke and cook until tender. (If you don't know how to prepare an artichoke there are instructional YouTube videos that demonstrate how. Alternatively, use frozen artichoke hearts)

IN a saucepan, add quinoa and two cups water. Bring to a boil, reduce heat, and cover. Simmer for 15 minutes.

IN a pan, heat olive oil and add tomatoes, cooked artichokes, and garlic, and stir-fry for 2–3 minutes. Dissolve yeast-free vegetable stock in ½ cup of water (check directions) and add to pan. Simmer on low heat for 2 more minutes, stirring occasionally. Finally, add the basil and the mint and season with cayenne pepper and salt. Pour the sauce over the cooked quinoa and serve immediately. Enjoy!

Alkalizing Raw Soup

This is definitely a highly energizing soup and a big favorite for those on a cleanse or detox program. It contains avocado, which is high in EFAs, and cucumber, which is well known for its cleansing properties. Feel free to play with the flavors by using the herbs and spices you enjoy!

½ avocado, diced

1 cup water

2 spring onions, chopped

½ red or green pepper, chopped

1 large cucumber, diced

2 cups baby spinach

½ clove fresh garlic, minced

juice of 1 lemon or lime

OPTIONAL: fresh minced cilantro, parsley, or basil leaves for taste.

OPTIONAL: ground coriander, dried parsley, ground cumin.

IN a blender or food processor, blend the avocado and water to form a light paste. Next add the other ingredients and continue to blend. Pour and sprinkle with the herbs of your choice. Enjoy!

IF you'd prefer a little warmth to the temperature of your soup, transfer to a saucepan and heat slowly until just warm and okay to touch.

Vibrant Avocado and Cucumber Soup

I know the thought of raw, lukewarm soup seems unappealing to many, but with loads of omega-3s, calcium, antioxidants, and too many vitamins to count, this soup is a great way to rebalance your body. So go on and give it a try!

1 avocado

1 small zucchini, chopped

2 ribs celery, chopped

2 cups baby spinach

1 cup fresh parsley

¼ cup fresh cilantro

½ cup green pepper, diced

¼ cup red onion, chopped

2 cloves fresh garlic, roughly chopped

¼ cup natural almonds, preferably soaked overnight and rinsed
(this makes them easier to blend and higher in enzymes)

1½ cups water

juice of 1 squeezed lemon

¼ tsp. Celtic sea salt

PLACE all the ingredients in the blender (except the sea salt) and blend to desired consistency. Transfer to a saucepan and gently warm over low heat until just warm enough to enjoy but not hot. Adjust seasoning to your liking. Serve and enjoy!

Skinny Jeans Tilapia Dish

Let's start with why tilapia is rock star among fat burning foods—protein. One serving of tilapia (4 oz.) has 29.5 grams of protein, which is more than 50 percent of your daily value of protein, meaning your body will be burning fat like crazy trying to process the protein! It is also high in vitamin B12, a nutrient that helps keep the body's nerve and blood cells healthy and helps make DNA, the genetic material in all cells. Vitamin B12 also helps prevent a type of anemia called megaloblastic anemia that makes people tired and weak. And with just 145 calories per serving, you can pair tilapia with a wide range of vegetables for a truly low-calorie and fat burning meal. Enjoy this delicious fish and be ready to slide into those skinny jeans in no time!

½ cup organic vegetable bouillon liquid or 1 cube

1 tsp. extra-virgin olive oil

sea salt to taste

4 (4-oz.) tilapia fillets

4-6 cherry tomatoes, halved

1 bunch parsley, minced

1 Tbsp. ground turmeric

15 natural almonds, chopped

½ cup apple cider vinegar

24 asparagus spears, steamed

PREHEAT oven to 350°F. In a large glass baking dish, pour in vegetable bouillon liquid, oil, and sea salt. Lay tilapia fillets in base of liquid and top with tomatoes and parsley. Sprinkle turmeric, almonds, and apple cider vinegar over top. Bake for 20–25 minutes or until flaky. Serve each with 6 steamed asparagus spears. Enjoy!

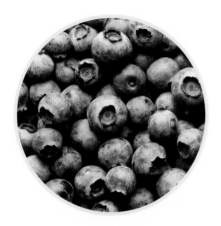

Raspberry Banana Smoothie

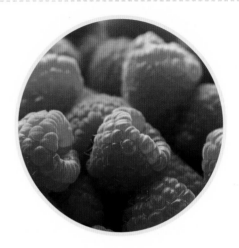

Sleepy Time Smoothie

Calcium rich sesame seeds, kale, and spinach make this smoothie the perfect nutritional lullaby. Also, a little protein before bed keeps your metabolism burning through the night. So relax, sip, and sleep!

1 cup water

¼ cup fresh or frozen blueberries

½ scoop iso—whey- or plant-based protein powder, your choice of flavor

1 Tbsp. ground or whole hemp seeds

⅓ cup natural sesame seeds

½ cup plain Greek or goat yogurt

1 tsp. organic dark honey

½ cup baby kale

½ cup baby spinach

> **COMBINE** all ingredients in a blender and blend until smooth. Pour and enjoy!

Loaded with vitamin C, antioxidants, and flavonoids to help boost your immune system, this bedtime smoothie will help your body heal as it sleeps so you wake feeling energized and in optimal health!

1 cup unsweetened plain almond or hemp milk

1 cup frozen raspberries

1 medium fresh banana

1 tsp. powdered glutamine

1 tsp. powdered magnesium

10 natural almonds, preferably soaked

1 tsp. natural nut butter

Optional: ½ scoop plant-based protein powder, your choice of flavor

> **COMBINE** all ingredients in a blender and blend until smooth. Pour and enjoy!

Sticky Cinnamon Toast

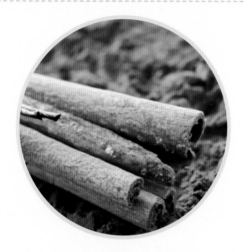

Raspberries offer a good dose of immune-boosting vitamin C, but they also contain calcium, which helps promote good sleep. They are also full of slow-digesting fiber, which means you will stay full all night without spiking your blood sugar levels before bed. The perfect bedtime treat!

1 slice gluten-free or yeast-free bread, toasted or plain

1 tsp. organic dark honey

1 tsp. ground cinnamon

⅓ cup fresh raspberries, crushed

> **SPREAD** all ingredients on plain or toasted bread. Enjoy with 1 cup chamomile, valerian root, or milk thistle tea (all of which promote sleep).

Slumber Supporting Oatmeal

As mentioned earlier, a high protein snack makes a great bedtime choice since it keeps your metabolism burning as you sleep. Furthermore, when your body is nutrient-depleted (like at the end of the day) it sends out signals to eat. Almonds are so nutrient rich that when consumed they stop these signals, thus preventing overeating, something that if done at bedtime severely impacts weight loss. Satisfy yourself properly before bed with this hearty oatmeal!

½ cup instant plain rolled oats

½ scoop iso—whey- or plant-based protein powder, your choice of flavor

10 natural almonds

> **COOK** oats according to package instructions. Stir in protein powder and almonds. Enjoy with 1 cup chamomile, valerian root, or milk thistle tea (all of which promote sleep).

Island Yogurt Parfait

Yogurt contains the amino-acid tryptophan, which studies show help you drift off into a peaceful slumber. Furthermore, studies show that carrying extra fat in your belly can negatively impact sleep. Coconut butter, nut butter, and cashews all offer a healthy dose of healthy omega-3s, which have been shown to reduce abdominal fat. Enjoy a little taste of the islands and make getting to sleep a breeze with this yogurt parfait.

1 cup organic plain yogurt

1 tsp. ground wheat germ

1 tsp. natural nut butter

1 tsp. coconut butter/oil

6 natural cashews

> **COMBINE** first four ingredients in a bowl and mix well. Sprinkle in cashews and serve. Enjoy with 1 cup chamomile, valerian root, or milk thistle tea (all of which promote sleep).

Cooling Nighttime Cucumber Juice

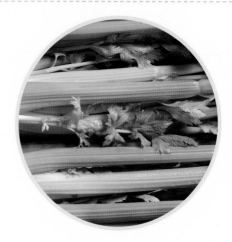

The last thing you want to do is consume a bunch of calories right before you go to sleep. This refreshing and filling juice will help stave off the bedtime munchies at next to no calories. Furthermore, the calcium in the spinach will help promote a restful sleep. Juice, sip, and snooze!

1 medium cucumber

2 cups baby spinach

2 ribs celery

2 ribs fennel

> **RUN** all ingredients through your juicer, pour, and enjoy!

WEEK ONE	DAY 1	DAY 2	DAY 3	DAY 4	DAY 5	DAY 6	DAY 7
MORNING CLEANSE DRINK	1 glass of distilled room temperature water mixed with ½ freshly squeezed lemon	1 glass of distilled room temperature water mixed with ½ freshly squeezed lemon	1 glass of distilled room temperature water mixed with ½ cup pure aloe vera juice	1 glass of distilled room temperature water mixed with ½ cup pure aloe vera juice	1 glass of distilled room temperature water mixed with ½ freshly squeezed lemon and 1 tsp. flax oil	1 glass of distilled room temperature water mixed with ½ freshly squeezed lemon and 1 tsp. flax oil	1 glass of distilled room temperature water mixed with ½ freshly squeezed lemon
BREAKFAST	Rise and Shine Shake (p. 113)	Choose 1 Breakfast Option	Calcium Smoothie (p. 118)	Choose 1 Breakfast Option	Lean Muscle Fruit n' Protein Pancakes (p. 123)	Choose 1 Smoothie Option	Protein-Packed Asparagus Omelette (p. 124)
MID-MORNING SNACK	We Got the "Beet" Juice	Weight Loss Tonic: Green Juice with Grapefruit (p. 133)	We Got the "Beet" Juice	Choose 1 Juice Option	Choose 1 Snack Option	We Got the "Beet" Juice (p. 129)	Choose 1 Snack Option
LUNCH	Cucumber Salad with Mint (p. 141)	Choose 1 Salad Option	Choose 1 Lunch Option	Choose 1 Salad Option	Choose 1 Lunch Option	Beet, Avocado, and Kelp Salad (p. 143)	Choose 1 Salad Option
MID-AFTERNOON SNACK	Choose 1 Snack Option	The Craving Crusher (p. 119)	Choose 1 Snack Option	Citrus Wheatgrass Juice (p. 125)	Choose 1 Juice Option	Choose 1 Snack Option	Tummy Warming Tonic (p. 128)
DINNER	Choose 1 Dinner or Entree Option	Cellulite Crusher Greens Salad (p. 144)	Choose 1 Entree Option	Choose 1 Entree Option	Choose 1 Dinner Option	Walnut, Fig, and Lentil Detox Salad (p. 146)	Choose 1 Entree Option
EVENING SNACK OPTIONAL	Sleepy Time Smoothie (p. 157)	Choose 1 Late Night Immunity Booster Option	Choose 1 Late Night Immunity Booster Option	Choose 1 Late Night Immunity Booster Option	Choose 1 Late Night Immunity Booster Option	Sleepy Time Smoothie (p. 157)	Choose 1 Late Night Immunity Booster Option

WEEK TWO	DAY 8	DAY 9	DAY 10	DAY 11	DAY 12	DAY 13	DAY 14
MORNING CLEANSE DRINK	1 glass of distilled room temperature water mixed with ½ freshly squeezed lemon & 1 tsp. probiotics	1 glass of distilled room temperature water mixed with ½ freshly squeezed lemon	1 glass of distilled room temperature water mixed with ½ cup pure aloe vera juice & 1 tsp. probiotics	1 glass of distilled room temperature water mixed with ½ cup pure aloe vera juice	1 glass of distilled room temperature water mixed with ½ freshly squeezed lemon and 1 tsp. flax oil	1 glass of distilled room temperature water mixed with ½ freshly squeezed lemon and 1 tsp. flax oil	1 glass of distilled room temperature water mixed with ½ freshly squeezed lemon& 1 tsp. omega-3
BREAKFAST	Cardio Apple and Beet Juice (p. 134)	Muscle-Building Spinach Juice (p. 135)	Weight Loss Tonic: Green Juice with Grapefruit (p. 133)	Sweet Cherry Almond Oatmeal (p. 123)	Weight Loss Tonic: Green Juice with Grapefruit (p. 133)	Choose 1 Breakfast Option	Choose 1 Breakfast Option
MID-MORNING SNACK	Wheatgrass shot (3-oz.)	Weight Loss Tonic: Green Juice with Grapefruit (p. 133)	Bone Builder Juice (p. 132)	½ cup plain yogurt mixed with 1 tsp. ground flax	1 brown rice cake topped with 1 tsp. natural nut butter and ground cinnamon	Workout Wonder Juice (p. 128)	Choose 1 Snack Option
LUNCH	Heart Booster Pomegranate Salad (p. 145)	Choose 1 Lunch or Salad Option	Choose 1 Lunch or Salad Option	Choose 1 Lunch or Salad Option	Beet, Avocado, and Kelp Salad (p. 143)	Choose 1 Salad Option	Choose 1 Salad Option
MID-AFTERNOON SNACK	Water Retention Juice (p. 132)	Water Retention Juice (p. 132)	½ cup plain yogurt mixed with 1 tsp. ground flax	Water Retention Juice (p. 132)	½ green apple 2 mini cucumbers	½ cup plain yogurt mixed with 1 tsp. ground flax	1 brown rice cake topped with 1 tsp. natural nut butter and ground cinnamon
DINNER	Choose 1 Dinner or Entree Option	Cellulite Crusher Greens Salad (p. 144)	Choose 1 Salad Option	Choose 1 Salad Option	Choose 1 Dinner Option	Walnut, Fig, and Lentil Detox Salad (p. 146)	Choose 1 Salad Option
EVENING SNACK OPTIONAL	Sleepy Time Smoothie (p. 157)	Choose 1 Late Night Immunity Booster Option	Choose 1 Late Night Immunity Booster Option	Cooling Nighttime Cucumber Juice (p. 159)	1 cup chamomile tea 1 cup celery sticks	Sleepy Time Smoothie (p. 157)	Choose 1 Late Night Immunity Booster Option

WEEK THREE	DAY 15	DAY 16	DAY 17	DAY 18	DAY 19	DAY 20	DAY 21
MORNING CLEANSE DRINK	1 glass of distilled room temperature water mixed with ½ freshly squeezed lemon & 1 tsp. probiotics	1 glass of distilled room temperature water mixed with½ freshly squeezed lemon & 1 tsp. probiotics	1 glass of distilled room temperature water mixed with 1 tsp. omega-3	1 glass of distilled room temperature water mixed with 1 tsp. omega-3	1 glass of distilled room temperature water mixed with ½ freshly squeezed lemon and 1 tsp. flax oil	1 glass of distilled room temperature water mixed with 1 tsp. probiotics &1 tsp. spirulina	1 glass of distilled room temperature water mixed with 1 tsp. probiotics & 1 tsp. spirulina
BREAKFAST	Choose 1 Salad Option	Choose 1 Salad Option	Weight Loss Tonic: Green Juice with Grapefruit (p. 133)	Choose 1 Breakfast Option	Choose 1 Juice Option	Choose 1 Breakfast Option	Choose 1 Breakfast Option
MID MORNING SNACK	1 cup fresh berries, plain	Weight Loss Tonic: Green Juice with Grapefruit (p. 133)	Bone Builder Juice (p. 132)	½ cup plain yogurt mixed with 1 tsp. ground flax	1 brown rice cake topped with 1 tsp. natural nut butter and ground cinnamon	Workout Wonder Juice (p. 128)	Choose 1 Juice Option
LUNCH	My Good Greens Salad (p. 146)	Choose 1 Lunch or Salad Option	Gut Happy Arugula Salad with Lemon Dill Dressing (p. 147)	Avocado Salad (p. 147)	Beet, Avocado, and Kelp Salad (p. 143)	Choose 1 Salad Option	Choose 1 Salad Option
MID AFTERNOON SNACK	Choose 1 Smoothie Option	½ banana 1 handful your choice natural nuts	The Craving Crusher (p. 119)	Choose 1 Snack Option	½ red apple 1 cup baby carrots and sliced fennel	½ cup plain yogurt mixed with 2 Tbsp. natural granola	1 brown rice cake topped with 1 tsp. natural nut butter and ground cinnamon
DINNER	Choose 1 Dinner or Entree Option	Cellulite Crusher Greens Salad (p. 144)	Amazing Mulligatawny Detox Soup (p. 152)	Amazing Mulligatawny Detox Soup (p. 152)	Choose 1 Dinner or Entree Option	Choose 1 Salad Option	Choose 1 Salad or Entree Option
EVENING SNACK OPTIONAL	Sleepy Time Smoothie (p. 157)	Cooling Nighttime Cucumber Juice (p. 159)	1 cup chamomile tea 1 cup celery sticks 10 natural almonds	Cooling Nighttime Cucumber Juice (p. 159)	Cooling Nighttime Cucumber Juice (p. 159)	Sleepy Time Smoothie (p. 157)	1 cup chamomile tea 1 cup celery sticks

THE 21-DAY DETOX
ACTIVE CLEANSE TRAINING PROGRAM

TOP TRAINING TIPS FROM EX-NFL ATHLETE AND CELEBRITY TRAINER MARC MEGNA

Marc has whipped some of the greatest professional athletes and hottest celebrities into shape. And now it's your turn with his exclusive beginner programs designed for you!

And as a special bonus, he's also offering you his top training tips to help you achieve a star-caliber body in no time!

1. Set goals. Always start any new fitness regimen by asking yourself what it is you want to achieve. Where do you want this training to take you? Having a clear goal is paramount to success. After all, you can't reach a destination if you don't know where you're going.

2. Keep a training journal. In order to reap maximum results from a program, you must chart your progress. Understanding where you are in your journey is the best way to keep moving forward and build on your hard work.

3. Get the best talent. You have made the decision to invest in yourself, so invest in a trainer who is experienced and has a quality certification. If you can't afford a trainer they will often be open to writing you a program at a more affordable cost.

4. Practice great form. To get the most out of your workout and to avoid injury, always make sure you are performing your exercise correctly and with control and detail. Safety first!

5. Lift those weights! Weight training has so many positive benefits and is a necessary component for any effective program. For starters, it increases the "good" cholesterol (HDL) while decreasing the "bad" cholesterol (LDL). It also reduces the risk of diseases such as diabetes, heart disease, cancer, and osteoporosis. It lowers blood pressure, reduces the effects and symptoms of premenstrual syndrome, and even staves off the common cold!

6. Push yourself! You want the best results, so make sure you are challenging yourself in training. If it's too easy you are not going to fully benefit from it, and then what has all that time you invested been worth? In terms of how challenging a workout should be, on a scale of 1 to 10, I like to always work at a 7 or an 8.

7. Train those legs! Your legs take you everywhere. They are your base and foundation, so give them the respect they deserve. Plus, no one wants chicken legs!

8. Commitment is key! Get used to the idea that you must be all in to get the results you want. Ask yourself the important question: Are you in? Or are you out? If you're in, commit and go for it!

9. Be consistent. As the old saying goes: repetition is the mother of learning. And that's never been truer than in regards to training. Only consistency in your program will give you the return on your time investment. Just remember to keep the challenge alive!

10. Give yourself a rest. The time you spend training is very important, but the 23 hours you spend outside the gym are paramount. You need time to sleep, rest, and recover!

For more information about Marc Megna, visit www.marcmegna.com.

MARC MEGNA'S
AT-HOME BEGINNER PROGRAM

» Reps—The number of times that you lift each weight or complete one movement

» Set—One completed series of reps after which you take a brief rest period

For example: To complete 3 sets of 5 reps, you would perform the exercise 5 times, then take a rest before repeating this process 2 more times.

DAY 1: QUADS AND BACK

Exercise	Week 1	Week 2
A1. Prisoner Squat (hands behind head) **Regression:** Hands on Hips Squat **Progression:** Overhead Squat (hands above head)	3 sets of 5 reps	3 sets of 8 reps
A2. Prone Towel Pull-Down	3 sets of 5 reps	3 sets of 8 reps
A3. Plank **Regression:** On Knees **Progression:** Feet Elevated	3 sets of 20 seconds	3 sets of 30 seconds
B1. Lateral Split Squat **Regression:** Lateral Squat **Progression:** Lateral Lunge	3 sets of 5 reps for each leg	3 sets of 8 reps for each leg
B2. Prone Ys	3 sets of 5 reps	3 sets of 8 reps
B3. Bird Dog	3 sets of 5 reps for each leg	3 sets of 8 reps for each leg

DAY 2: HAMSTRINGS, GLUTES, CHEST, AND SHOULDERS

Exercise	Week 1	Week 2
A1. Prisoner Hip Hinge **Regression:** Hands on Hips Hip Hinge **Progression:** Overhead Hip Hinge (hands above head)	3 sets of 5 reps	3 sets of 8 reps
A2. Push-Up **Regression:** Hands Elevated **Progression:** Feet Elevated	3 sets of 5 reps	3 sets of 8 reps
A3. Reverse Fly	3 sets of 5 reps	3 sets of 8 reps
B1. Hip Press **Regression:** Hip Bridge for 10 seconds **Progression:** Single Leg Hip Press	3 sets of 5 reps	3 sets of 8 reps
B2. Standing Thumbs Up Front and Lateral Raise	3 sets of 5 reps for each leg	3 sets of 8 reps for each leg
B3. Arms at Side Straight Leg Sit-Up	3 sets of 8 reps	3 sets of 10 reps

DAY 3: QUADS, CALVES, AND BACK

Exercise	Week 1	Week 2
A1. Split Squat **Regression:** Bottoms Up Split Squat **Progression:** Front Lunge	3 sets of 5 reps for each leg	3 sets of 8 reps for each leg
A2. Tall Kneeling Towel Row	3 sets of 5 reps	3 sets of 8 reps
A3. Prone Walk-Out	3 sets of 5 reps	3 sets of 8 reps
B1. Standing Calf Press **Regression:** Wall Calf Press **Progression:** Single Leg Standing Calf Press	3 sets of 8 reps	3 sets of 10 reps
B2. Prone Ts	3 sets of 5 reps	3 sets of 8 reps
B3. Prisoner Good Morning	3 sets of 5 reps	3 sets of 8 reps

DAY 4: HAMSTRINGS, GLUTES, CHEST, AND SHOULDERS

Exercise	Week 1	Week 2
A1. Prisoner Reverse Lunge **Regression:** Hands on Hips Reverse Lunge **Progression:** Overhead Reverse Lunge (hands above head)	3 sets of 5 reps for each leg	3 sets of 8 reps for each leg
A2. Push-Up **Regression:** Hands Elevated **Progression:** Feet Elevated	3 sets of 5 reps	3 sets of 8 reps
A3. Prone Front Raise	3 sets of 5 reps	3 sets of 8 reps
B1. Single Leg Reaching Deadlift **Regression:** Wall Single Leg Deadlift **Progression:** Prisoner Single Leg Deadlift	3 sets of 5 reps for each leg	3 sets of 8 reps for each leg
B2. Shoulder Walk-Out	3 sets of 5 reps	3 sets of 8 reps
B3. Arms Crossed at Chest Straight Leg Sit-Up	3 sets of 5 reps	3 sets of 8 reps

MARC MEGNA'S
IN-THE-GYM BEGINNER PROGRAM

» Reps—The number of times that you lift each weight or complete one movement

» Set—One completed series of reps after which you take a brief rest period

For example: To complete 3 sets of 5 reps, you would perform the exercise 5 times, then take a rest before repeating this process 2 more times.

DAY 1: LEGS AND BACK

Exercise	Week 1	Week 2
A1. Dumbbell or Kettlebell Goblet Squat	3 sets of 5 reps	3 sets of 8 reps
A2. Neutral Grip Chin-Up (band assisted if necessary)	3 sets of 5 reps	3 sets of 8 reps
A3. Plank	3 sets of 20 seconds	3 sets of 30 seconds
B1. Single Dumbbell or Kettlebell Reverse Lunge	3 sets of 5 reps for each leg	3 sets of 8 reps for each leg
B2. Suspension Row	3 sets of 5 reps	3 sets of 8 reps
B3. Tall Kneeling Belly Press	3 sets of 5 reps on each side	3 sets of 8 reps on each side

DAY 2: CHEST, SHOULDERS, AND ARMS

Exercise	Week 1	Week 2
A1. Dumbbell Chest Press	3 sets of 5 reps	3 sets of 8 reps
A2. Barbell Biceps Curl	3 sets of 5 reps	3 sets of 8 reps
A3. Prone Front Raise	3 sets of reps on each side	3 sets of 8 reps on each side
B1. Half Kneeling Dumbbell Overhead Press	3 sets of 5 reps	3 sets of 8 reps
B2. Cable Triceps Press-down	3 sets of 5 reps	3 sets of 8 reps
B3. Bench Reverse Hyper	3 sets of 8 reps	3 sets of 10 reps

DAY 3: LEGS AND BACK

Exercise	Week 1	Week 2
A1. Dumbbell or Kettlebell Split Squat	3 sets of 5 reps for each leg	3 sets of 8 reps for each leg
A2. Half Kneeling Cable Row	3 sets of 5 reps for each arm	3 sets of 8 reps for each arm
A3. Stability Ball Roll-Out	3 sets of 8 reps	3 sets of 10 reps
B1. Kettlebell or Dumbbell Deadlift	3 sets of 5 reps	3 sets of 8 reps
B2. Dumbbell Bent-Over Row	3 sets of 5 reps for each arm	3 sets of 8 reps for each arm
B3. Side Plank	3 sets of 15 seconds on each side	3 sets of 20 seconds on each side

Exercise	Week 1	Week 2
A1. Incline Dumbbell Chest Press	3 sets of 5 reps	3 sets of 8 reps
A2. Half Kneeling Rope Cable Face Pull	3 sets of 5 reps	3 sets of 8 reps
A3. Prone Walk-Out	3 sets of 5 reps	3 sets of 8 reps
B1. Dumbbell Curl and Press	3 sets of 5 reps	3 sets of 8 reps
B2. Diamond Push-Ups	3 sets of 5 reps	3 sets of 8 reps
B3. Dumbbell or Kettlebell Farmer Carry	3 sets of 20 steps	3 sets of 30 steps

AT-HOME BEGINNER EXERCISE PLAN APPENDIX

PRISONER SQUAT

A) Start by standing as tall as you can with your feet spread shoulder-width apart, placing your fingers on the back of your head (as if you had just been arrested).

B) Lower your body as far as you can by pushing your hips back and bending your knees. The tops of your thighs should be parallel to the floor. Pause for one second, then slowly push yourself back to the starting position.

Note: Keep your weight on your heels, not your toes, for the entire movement. Your knees should stay over the centers of your feet as you squat, and your torso should stay as upright as possible.

Regression: Hands on Hips Squat—perform the above movements with your hands on your hips.

Progression: Overhead Squat—perform the above movement with your hands above your head.

PRONE TOWEL PULL-DOWN

A) Start by lying down on your stomach and slightly raise your chest. Grab a towel with both hands above your head. Pull the towel apart and extend your arms out straight.

B) Pull the towel toward your chest while bending elbows, then return to starting position.

PLANK

A) Starting by lying down on your stomach, resting your body on your forearms with your palms flat on the floor. Double check that your shoulders are aligned directly over your elbows. Make sure that your legs are straight behind you with your ankles, knees, and thighs touching.

B) In a push-up motion, raise your body off the floor, supporting your weight on your forearms and your toes. You should have a straight line from your feet to your head. Keep your abdominal muscles engaged and do not let your stomach drop or allow for your hips to rise up. To avoid letting your hips or butt rise up, tilt your pelvis toward the floor. Remember to breath. Take slow inhales and exhale steadily.

C) To begin, hold this position for 20 seconds, keeping your abs engaged and your body in a straight line. Repeat 3–5 times.

Regression: Lower your knees to the ground, so instead of balancing on your toes you are in a modified plank position with your lower body supported by your knees.

Progression: Alternate lifting one foot off the ground as you hold your plank.

LATERAL SPLIT SQUAT

A) Start in a standing position and spread your legs as far apart as you comfortably can. With your arms extended straight in front of you, shift weight to one leg and slowly sit back. Emphasize moving hips backward rather than knees forward. Switch to opposite side.

B) Start slowly moving back and forth, increasing speed at your own pace to make sure the motion doesn't shorten.

Regression: Lateral Squat—Standing with your feet wider than shoulder width apart, shift your hips to the left and down by bending your left knee and keeping your right leg straight. Your feet should be straight ahead and flat on the ground. Push through your left hip, returning to the starting position. Alternate sides and repeat for the prescribed number of repetitions.

Progression: Lateral Lunge—Start by standing with your feet shoulder width apart, hands on hips. Step out to the right and shift your body weight over your right leg, squatting to a 90 degree angle at the right knee. Try to sit down with your butt, keeping your back as upright as possible. Push off and bring your right leg back to center to complete one rep. Finish all reps on this side and repeat on the left side to complete one set.

PRONE Y

A) Start by lying on your stomach with your arms above your head. Slowly lift your arms up in a diagonal direction so that your shoulder blades pinch back behind you and you are making the letter "Y" with your body.

B) Hold this "Y" position for one to two seconds then slowly lower back down to the starting position.

BIRD DOG

A) Start by kneeling on the floor on all fours with your hands firmly placed about shoulder width apart.

B) Brace the abdominals, and practice lifting one hand and the opposite knee just clear of the floor while balancing on the other hand and knee. Half an inch will do until you get the idea of it.

C) When you're ready to do the complete exercise, point the arm out straight in front and extend the opposite leg to the rear. Hold for 10 seconds then return to hands and knees to the ground in the starting position.

DAY 2

PRISONER HIP HINGE

A) Start by standing with your feet shoulder-width apart, toes pointed forward or slightly outward. Place your hands on the back of your head just as you did in the prisoner squat exercise.

B) Gently exhale. Shift your weight onto your heels, push your hips back, and hinge forward at the hips until your torso is midway between vertical and parallel to the floor. Allow only slight bending at the knees throughout this movement.

C) Gently inhale. Contract your glutes. Push your hips forward and upward, slowly returning to upright.

Regression: Hands on Hips Squat—perform the above movements with your hands on your hips.

Progression: Overhead Squat—perform the above movement with your hands above your head.

PUSH-UP

A) Start by getting into a plank position with your hands planted directly under the shoulders (slightly wider than shoulder width apart). Ground the toes into the floor to stabilize the bottom half of the body. Engage the abs and back so the body is neutral.

B) Begin to lower the body—back flat, eyes focused about three feet in front of you to keep a neutral neck—until the chest nearly touches the floor. Don't let the butt dip or stick out at any point during the move; the body should remain flat from head to toe all the way through the movement. Draw the shoulder blades back and down, while keeping the elbows tucked close to the body, so the upper arms form a 45-degree angle at the bottom of the push-up position.

C) Keeping the core engaged, exhale as you push back to the start position.

Regression: perform the above movements with your hands elevated, such facing upward with your hands on a bench or flight of stairs.

Progression: perform the above movement with your feet elevated, such facing downward on a bench or flight of stairs.

REVERSE FLY

A) Start by holding a pair of dumbbells at your side, stand with your feet hip-width apart and your knees bent. Bend forward at the hips and let your arms hang straight down from your shoulders, palms facing inwards. Raise both arms out to the sides as you squeeze your shoulder blades together.

B) Slowly lower arms back down, returning to starting position.

HIP PRESS

A) Start lying down face up on the floor with your knees bent and your feet flat. Place your arms out to your sides at 45-degree angles, your palms facing up. Brace your core—as if you're about to be punched in the gut—and hold it that way.

B) Squeeze your glutes tightly and raise your hips until your body forms a straight line from your shoulders to your knees. Pause for up to 5 seconds in the up position—as you continue to squeeze your glutes—then lower your body back to the starting position.

Regression: Perform step A and hold position for 10 seconds instead of moving to step B.

Progression: Single Leg Hip Press—perform the hip press with one leg on the ground and the other extended out. Alternate between legs.

STANDING THUMBS UP FRONT LATERAL RAISE

A) Start standing with your feet shoulder-width apart, back straight, knees slightly bent, and your arms resting on your thighs.

B) Lift your arms up shoulder height with your thumbs pointing up toward the ceiling. Return to starting position.

Progression: Add light to medium heavy dumbbells.

ARMS AT SIDE STRAIGHT LEG SIT-UP

A) Start lying down on the floor with your legs straight out in front of you and your arms at your sides. Contract your abdominals to pull yourself up into a sitting position.

B) Slowly lower yourself back down to starting position.

SPLIT SQUAT

A) Start in a standing position with one foot forward and other foot behind. Squat down by flexing the knee and hip of front leg. Allow heel of rear foot to rise up while knee of rear leg bends slightly until it almost makes contact with floor.

B) Return to original standing position by extending hip and knee of forward leg. Repeat. Continue with opposite leg.

Regression: Bottoms Up Split Squat—Perform the above movement with one foot resting on a chair or bench.

Progression: Front lunge—Start in a standing position, feet hip-width apart and your arms relaxed at your sides. Take a big step forward with your right leg then slowly bend your front knee so that it is at a 90 degree angle with the floor and your back knee almost touches the floor. Keeping your weight on your front (right) heel, contract your front (right) quad along with your hamstrings and glutes to push yourself back up to the starting position. Focus on doing each rep slowly and steadily to avoid knee strain.

TALL KNEELING TOWEL ROW

A) Start down on one knee and grab the ends of your towel with both hands, pulling it taught and palms facing down. If you are kneeling on your right knee, you will be working with the right arm, and vice versa.

B) Engage your core and pull the one end of the towel into your body (in a rowing motion), keeping your torso straight.

B) Slowly return back to starting position. Repeat all reps on one side, and then switch.

PRONE WALK-OUT

A) Begin on all fours with only your hands and toes touching the ground (so your body is in a "V" shape). With your core engaged, slowly walk your hands forward without moving your feet or toes until you are in a plank position.

B) With your core still engaged, walk your hands back to where you began without losing balance.

STANDING CALF PRESS

A) Position toes and balls of feet on a step (your staircase will work) with arches and heels extending off.

B) Raise your heels by extending your ankles as high as possible (like you're in a pair of very high heels). Then lower heels by bending ankle until calf is stretched. Repeat.

Regression: Wall Calf Press—Stand 6–12 inches away from a wall with your feet hip-width apart and toes facing forward. Place your hands on the wall, shoulder height. Slowly rise up on to your toes, lifting your heels off the floor while keeping your knees straight. Use your hands on the wall to support your balance. Hold the raised position briefly. Inhale and slowly lower your heels back to the floor.

PRONE TS

A) Start lying face down on the ground with your arms extended out in a "T" position. Slowly lift your arms upward and pinch your shoulder blade back toward your spine.

PRISONER GOOD MORNING

A) Start by standing with your feet hip-width apart and pointing straight ahead and place your hands behind your head. Draw your navel in toward your spine, and contract your abdominals to stabilize your spine. Keep your legs straight and your back

Progression: Single Leg Standing Calf Press—Perform the same movement as the regular Standing Calf Press while lifting one leg to rear, bending your knee so you are balancing on one leg as you perform the exercise. Do a complete set on one leg, then switch.

B) Hold this position for 1–2 seconds, and then slowly lower back to the starting position.

flat as you hinge forward at your hips, and lower your torso parallel to the floor. Pause for one count.

B) Return to the starting position without releasing your abdominals.

DAY 4

PRISONER REVERSE LUNGE

A) Start by standing with your feet shoulder-width apart and clasp your hands behind your head. Keep your elbows pulled back and your shoulder blades pulled together to work the upper back. Step forward with one leg, taking a slightly larger than normal step. Be sure to keep your right toe on the ground and use it to help keep your balance, and also bend your right knee. Continue to lower your body until your front thigh is parallel to the ground, keeping your upper body upright throughout the entire movement.

B) Push with your front leg to return to the starting position and swap legs.

Regression: Hands on Hips Reverse Lunge—perform the above movement with your hands on your hips instead of behind your head.

Progression: Overhead Reverse Lunge—perform the above movement with your hands stretched above your head instead of behind your head.

PRONE FRONT RAISE

A) Start lying down on a bench with a dumbbell in each hand and your arms hanging straight down toward the floor (if you don't have access to a bench, your bed will do). Keeping a slight bend in your elbows, exhale as you lift the dumbbells up in front of you until they are at head height.

B) Hold for one second, then slowly lower back down to starting position.

Regression: Perform exercise one arm at a time.

SINGLE LEG REACHING DEADLIFT

A) Start in a standing position with your arms directly above your head. One knee should be elevated to a 90-degree angle. Sweep your hands down toward the floor and extend the lifted leg so it is straight.

B) Making sure your back is straight, hold the position for a couple of seconds before returning to the starting position.

Regression: Wall Single Leg Deadlift—perform the above movement with the side of your body opposite the leg you are lifting up against a wall for balance.

Progression: Prisoner Single Leg Deadlift—perform the traditional Single Leg Reaching Deadlift with your hands clasped behind your head instead of reaching in front.

SHOULDER WALKOUT

A) Start bent over with your hands and feet on the ground in a "V" position. Engage your core and slowly walk your hands out away from your feet until you are in a plank position.

B) Perform one push-up, and then slowly walk your hands back to starting position.

ARMS CROSSED AT CHEST STRAIGHT LEG SIT-UP

A) Start lying on your back with your arms crossed on your chest and one leg extended outward (the other is bent at a 90 degree angle).

B) Engage your core and slowly lift your shoulders off the ground. Hold for 1 second, then slowly lower back to starting position. Finish one complete set, then switch legs.

IN-THE-GYM BEGINNER EXERCISE PLAN APPENDIX

DAY 1

DUMBBELL KETTLEBELL GOBLET SQUAT

A) Start standing with your feet shoulder-width apart and the dumbbell or kettlebell against your chest. Squat down as low as you can while pushing your butt out (like you're sitting down on a chair).

B) Hold the squat position for one second then rise back, squeezing your glutes, to the starting position.

NEUTRAL GRIP CHIN-UP

A) Start standing in front of the bar and grab the parallel handles of the chin-up station so that your palms are facing each other.

B) Pull your chest to the level of the bars, pause, then slowly lower your body back to a dead hang.

PLANK

A) Start in a push-up position, resting your body on your forearms with your palms flat on the floor. Double check that your shoulders are aligned directly over your elbows. Make sure that your legs are straight behind you with your ankles, knee, and thighs touching.

B) In a push-up motion, raise your body off the floor, supporting your weight on your forearms and your toes. You should have a straight line from your feet to your head. Keep your abdominal muscles engaged and do not let your stomach drop or allow your hips to rise up. To avoid letting your hips or buttock rise up, tilt your pelvis toward the floor. Remember to breath. Take slow inhales and exhale steadily.

C) To begin, hold this position for 20 seconds, keeping your abs engaged and your body in a straight line. Repeat 3–5 times.

SINGLE DUMBBELL OR KETTLEBELL REVERSE LUNGE

A) Start standing with your feet shoulder width apart and hold a dumbbell or kettlebell vertically in front of your chest, cupping one end of the dumbbell with both hands or holding the horns of the kettlebell. Keep your elbows pointed toward the floor and step back with your right leg, balancing on the ball of your foot. Bend your knees and lower yourself toward the floor. Your lower left leg should be perpendicular to the floor with your left knee aligned over your ankle. Your right knee should drop to within a couple of inches of the floor.

B) Pause for 1 second and then stand back up, pushing through the heel of your left leg and pulling your right leg back into a standing position. Complete all repetitions on one leg first, or alternate sides, with one complete lunge on each side counting as one rep.

SUSPENSION ROW

A) Attach a pair of straps with handles to a secure bar so that the handles are about 3 feet off the floor. Grab the handles and place your hands shoulder-width apart.

B) Start the movement by pulling your shoulder blades back, then continue the pull with your arms to lift your chest to the handles. Pause, then slowly lower your body back to the starting position.

TALL KNEELING BELLY PRESS

A) Start by attaching a D-handle at chest height to a cable machine. Begin in a kneeling position with your back tall and your core engaged, holding the handle with both hands. Slowly press your arms in front of you until they're straight.

B) Without letting your body rotate, hold the position for 1 second, and then slowly bring them back to your chest. When all reps are completed on one side, turn and perform on the other side.

DUMBBELL CHEST PRESS

A) Start by lying down on a bench with a dumbbell in each hand and your feet flat on the floor. You can rest your feet up on the bench if it's more comfortable. Push the dumbbells up so that your arms are directly over your shoulders and your palms are up. Slowly lower the dumbbells down and a little to the side until your elbows are slightly below your shoulders.

B) Slowly push the weights back up with control, taking care not to lock your elbows or allow your shoulder blades to rise off the bench. Repeat.

BARBELL BICEP CURL

A) Start standing with feet shoulder width apart and grasp the bar, holding on with an underhand grip. With elbows to side, raise the bar until forearms are vertical.

B) Slowly lower the bar back down with control until your arms are fully extended. Repeat.

PRONE FRONT RAISE

A) Start lying stomach down on a bench with a dumbbell in each hand and your arms hanging straight down toward the floor, hands under your shoulders with palms facing behind you. Keeping a slight bend in your elbows, exhale as your lift the dumbbells up in front of you until they are at head height.

B) Inhale as you lower the dumbbells back to starting position.

Regression: Perform exercise one arm at a time.

HALF KNEELING OVERHEAD PRESS

A) Start with one knee on the ground and the other leg bent in front at a 45-degree angle, holding a pair of dumbbells at your shoulders, palms facing forward. Keeping your legs and torso stable, press the weights overhead.

B) Slowly lower the weights back down to the starting position. Repeat.

CABLE TRICEPS PRESS-DOWN

A) Start in a standing position, feet shoulder-width apart, facing a high pulley machine. Grasp the cable attachment with an overhand narrow grip and position your elbows to side. Extend arms downward, pulling cable handle to hip level.

B) Slowly bring your arms back up until your forearm is close to your upper arm. Repeat.

BENCH REVERSE HYPER

A) Start lying down on a bench with your hips on the edge and your legs straight, toes resting on the floor. Raise your legs as high as possible until your body is in a straight line.

B) Lower legs back down to original position. Repeat.

DAY 3

DUMBBELL OR KETTLEBELL SPLIT SQUAT

A) Start by finding a bench or other suitable object roughly one to two feet high. Grasp a dumbbell or kettlebell with a goblet grip—where both hands grasp the top portion of a dumbbell in an upward motion or the horns of the kettlebell. Plant your working foot one stride's length in front of the bench and place the top of your stabilizing foot flat on the bench.

B) Bracing through your core, descend to a point just before your knee touches the floor. Keep the knee in line with the toe and do not bend forward.

C) Slowly raise yourself back up into starting position by pushing through your front heel. Repeat.

HALF KNEELING CABLE ROW

A) Start down on one knee in front of the cable machine, about 3 feet away. Grab the cable handle with both hands, palms facing in. Engage your core and pull the handle into your body and rotate the palms of your hands upward.

B) Slowly return back to starting position. Repeat.

STABILITY BALL ROLL-OUT

A) Start kneeling in front of a stability ball with your knees hip-width apart, then place your forearms on the ball, hands in loose fists. Keeping your back flat, brace your core and slowly roll the ball away from you by straightening your arms; extend as far as you can without allowing your hips to drop.

B) Pause for one second, then bend your elbows to roll the ball back to starting position. Repeat.

DUMBBELL OR KETTLEBELL DEADLIFT

A) Start standing with your feet about hip-width apart and a kettlebell or dumbbells on the floor in front of you. Engage your core and bend the knees, keeping your back flat as you lower down into a squat to pick up the weight. Squat as low as you can, keeping the hips back and the knees behind the toes, and make sure the abs are braced.

B) Pick up the weight and stand up, using the power of your legs to push back to start. Repeat.

DUMBBELL BENT-OVER ROW

A) Start by kneeling over the side of a bench, placing one knee and the hand of the supporting arm on the bench. Position foot of opposite leg slightly back to side and grasp the dumbbell from the floor.

B) Pull the dumbbell up to your side until it makes contact with your ribs or until upper arm is just beyond horizontal.

C) Return to starting position by lowering your arm until arm is extended and shoulder is stretched downward. Perform all reps on that side, then switch.

SIDE PLANK

A) Start by lying on your left side with your knees straight. Prop your upper body up on your left elbow and forearm. Raise your hips until your body forms a straight line from your ankles to your shoulders. Hold this position for 30 seconds. Turn around so that you're lying on your right side and repeat.

DAY 4

INCLINE DUMBBELL CHEST PRESS

A) Start by sitting down on an inclining bench with dumbbells resting on your lower thighs. Bring the weights up to your shoulders and lean back. Position the dumbbells to the sides of your chest with your upper arm under each dumbbell.

B) Press the dumbbells up with elbows to the side until your arms are extended.

C) Lower weights back down to the sides of your upper chest until slight stretch is felt in your chest or shoulders. Repeat.

HALF KNEELING ROPE CABLE FACE PULL

A) Start by kneeling down at the cable station so that your outside knee is on the floor but your inside knee is bent 90 degrees, with your inside foot flat on the floor. Your left side should face the weight stack.

B) With both hands, grasp the rope with an overhand grip at arm's length, just in front of your left shoulder, keeping your hands about 18 inches apart. Your shoulders should be turned toward the rope, but your belly button should be pointing forward. Your torso should be upright. Allow your torso to rotate as you pull the rope past your outside hip. Don't round your lower back and keep your arms straight and your core braced. Complete the prescribed number of repetitions to your right side, and then do the same number with your right side facing the stack, pulling toward your left.

PRONE WALK-OUT

A) Begin on all fours with only your hands and toes touching the ground (your body should be in a "V" position). With your core engaged, slowly walk your hands forward without moving your feet or toes until you are in a plank position.

B) With your core still engaged, walk your hands back to starting position without losing balance.

DUMBBELL CURL AND PRESS

A) Start by standing with your feet shoulder width apart holding a pair of dumbbells at your sides. Curl the weights up, rotating your palms so they're facing your shoulders.

B) Next press the weights over your head, again rotating as you go so your palms face forward at the top of the movement.

C) Reverse the movement to return to starting position. Repeat.

DIAMOND PUSH-UPS

A) Start by getting into a regular push-up position, then move both of your hands under your chest (breast area) and make a pyramid-like shape with your hands. Your pointing fingers should touch and your thumb should touch on the bottom.

B) Begin to lower the body—back flat, eyes focused about three feet in front of you to keep a neutral neck—until the chest nearly touches the floor. Don't let the butt dip or stick out at any point during the move; the body should remain flat from head to toe all the way through the movement. Draw the shoulder blades back and down while keeping the elbows tucked close to the body so the upper arms form a 45-degree angle at the bottom of the push-up position.

C) Keeping the core engaged, exhale as you push back to the start position.

DUMBBELL OR KETTLEBELL FARMER CARRY

A) Start by placing the weights you will be using (dumbbells or kettlebell) on each side of your body. Bend down and grab the weight, keeping back straight, head forward, and arms extended. Stand up with the weight just as if you are performing a deadlift.

B) Begin to walk forward with the weight, keeping your head forward and shoulders back at all times.

C) Continue walking until you complete your prescribed amount of steps. Rest and repeat for the prescribed number of walks.

ADELE'S 21-DAY DETOX ACTION PLAN AND GOAL SETTING TEMPLATE

Goal	Actions Required	Resources Needed	Target Date of Completion	Status/ Comments

[RECIPE INDEX]

3 3138 00617 0954

613 FR

All affirmations inspired by: http://www.vitalaffirmations.com

"Bowel Motions," Better Health Channel, last modified August 2011, accessed January 16, 2013, http://www.betterhealth.vic.gov.au/bhcv2/bhcarticles.nsf/pages/Bowel_motions.

Carr, Kriss. Crazy Sexy Diet (Globe Pequot Press, 2011).

Edgar, Julie. "Types of Teas and Their Health Benefits," WebMD, accessed January 23, 2013, http://www.webmd.com/diet/features/tea-types-and-their-health-benefits.

Ehrlich, Caryl. "Four Stages of Breaking a Food Addiction" Psych Central (2005), http://psychcentral.com/library/food_stages.htm. Accessed February 25, 2013.

Edward Esko. "A Guide to the Health Benefits of Green Tea," The Preventive Medicine Center, accessed January 25, 2013, http://www.thepmc.org/2009/12/library-health-benefits-of-green-tea/.

"Food Addicts Anonymous," accessed February 25, 2013, http://www.foodaddictsanonymous.org.

Haiken, Melanie. "Dangerous Beauty: 5 Scariest Beauty Products," Forbes, last modified March 12, 2012, accessed January 23, 2013, http://www.forbes.com/sites/melaniehaiken/2012/03/12/dangerous-beauty-top-5-contaminated-beauty-products/.

"Heart & Stroke Health Check: Nutrient Standards for Sugar," Heart and Stroke Foundation, accessed February 15, 2013, http://www.heartandstroke.com/site/c.ikIQLcMWJtE/b.4391503/k.B3D/Health_Check_nutrient_standards_for_sugar.htm.

Joshi, Nish. Joshi's Alkaline Diet (Hodder & Stoughton, 2013).

Kresser, Chris. "Why Grass-Fed Trumps Grain-Fed," Chris Kresser: Let's Take Back Your Health, accessed January 15, 2013, http://chriskresser.com/why-grass-fed-trumps-grain-fed.

Langlois, Kellie and Garriguet, Didier. "Sugar Consumption Among Canadians of All Ages," Statistics Canada, accessed February 5, 2013, http://www.statcan.gc.ca/pub/82-003-x/2011003/article/11540-eng.htm.

Lipman, Frank, M.D. "20 Ways to 'Detox' Your Home" The Huffington Post (2010), accessed January 23, 2013, http://www.huffingtonpost.com/dr-frank-lipman/20-ways-to-detox-yourhom_b_682615.html.

Nordqvist, Christian. "What is Acupuncture? What Are the Benefits of Acupuncture?" Medical News Today, last modified July 6, 2009, accessed March 3, 2013, http://www.medicalnewstoday.com/articles/156488.php.

Orenstein, Beth W. "How to Know If You're Lactose Intolerant," Everyday Health, accessed February 13, 2013, http://www.everydayhealth.com/digestive-health/lactose-intolerance.aspx.

"Protein for Active Canadians," Canadian Society for Exercise Physiology (2011), accessed February 2, 2013, http://www.csep.ca/CMFiles/publications/dfc/Protein_booklet_e.pdf.

"Raw Food Life," accessed February 1, 2013, http://www.rawfoodlife.com.

Sword, Rosemary K.M. "Toxic Relationships" Psychology Today (2013), accessed January 23, 2013, http://www.psychologytoday.com/blog/the-time-cure/201308/toxic-relationships.

Weil, Andrew, M.D. "Q & A Section," WEILTM Andrew Weil, M.D., last modified May 15, 2006, accessed January 23, 2013, http://www.drweil.com/drw/u/QAA365093/Chia-for-Health.html.

Weil, Andrew, M.D., "Q & A Section," WEILTM Andrew Weil, M.D., last modified July 9, 2009, accessed January 23, 2013, http://www.drweil.com/drw/u/QAA400584/High-on-Hemp-Milk.html.

"Why Is Sleep Important?" National Heart, Lung, and Blood Institute, last modified February 22, 2012, accessed February 13, 2013, http://www.nhlbi.nih.gov/health/health-topics/topics/sdd/why.html.

"Your Digestive System and How It Works," International Foundation for Functional Gastrointestinal Disorders, last modified April 22, 2014, accessed April 30, 2014, http://www.iffgd.org/site/gi-disorders/digestive-system.

Logan Hocking County
District Library
230 East Main Street
Logan, Ohio 43138